Sex Games for Couples

Naughty and Fun Sex Games to Awaken Sexiness, Seduction and Rekindle the Spark in Your Relationship

Riley Ashwood

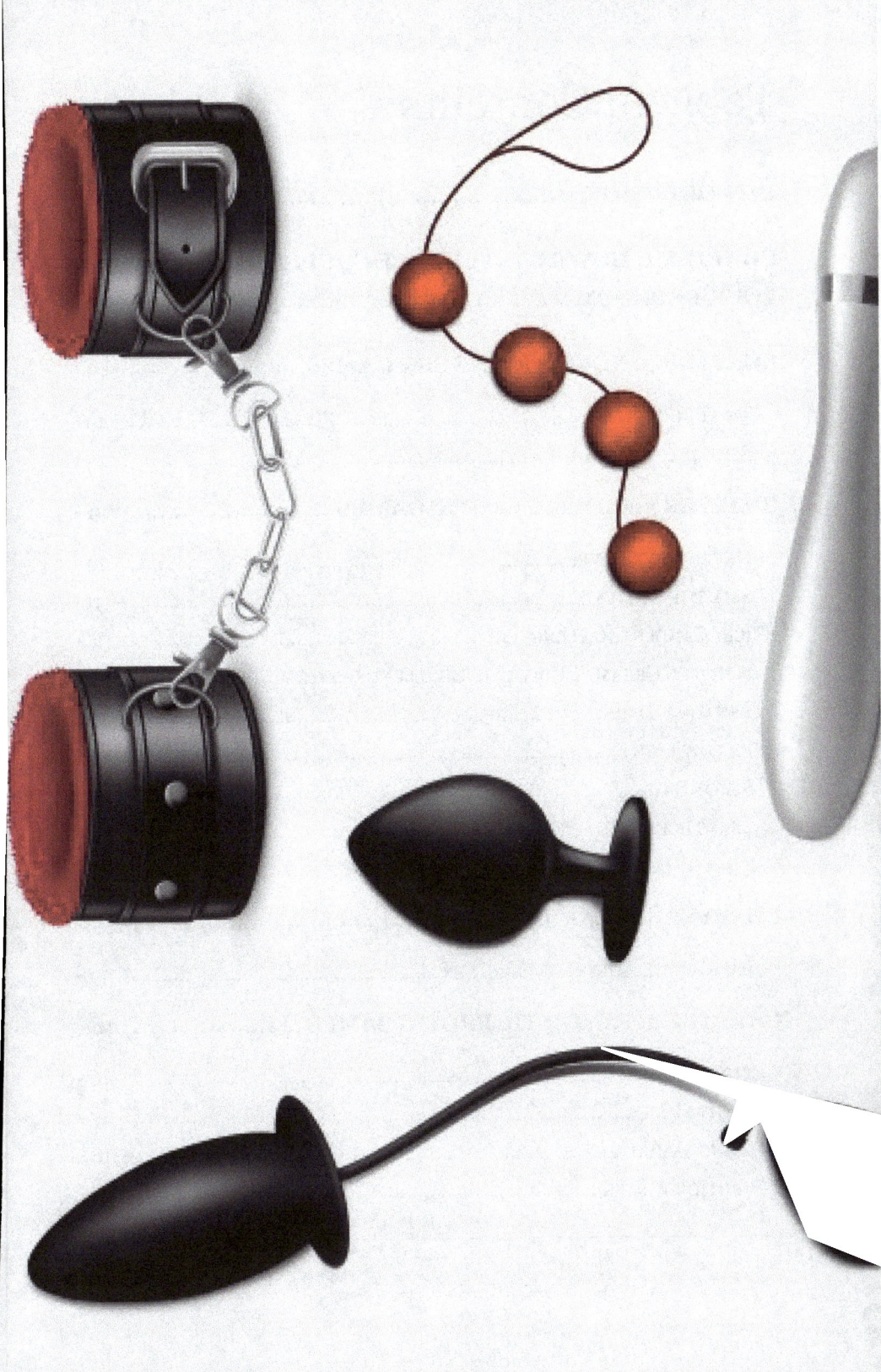

Table of Contents

Introduction

Having intercourse is a sexual action that communicates the affection, enthusiasm, care and other solid sentiments you have for someone else. It is a delightful and passionate experience that can bring two individuals ever nearer together. Lovemaking ought to be the point at which you and your partner both feel loose, secure and upbeat. In spite of the fact that this might be valid, numerous individuals worry when the idea of having intercourse rings a bell since they are making a decent attempt to make sense of what the correct method to have intercourse is.

Such a significant number of ladies can't accomplish their pleasure-potential on the grounds that their man has a constrained perspective on what lovemaking is. (On the off chance that you are straight, gay, single, wedded, strange, poly, trans... it's all great... this lovemaking strategy can be altered by you to your sexual fulfillment.)

Sex goes past the snapshot of infiltration. All that you're doing isn't paving the way to intercourse. The entire lovemaking background can be orgasmic when you realize how to bring a lady into her sexual personality state and afterward give her stacking, growing orgasmic joy. Prior to making that move to have intercourse, it is significant that you connect with yourself first. What is simply the status of your regard? Having high and sound confidence has a major effect on your lovemaking exhibitions. On the off chance that there is something in particular about yourself that makes you shaky, set an objective on overcoming that uncertainty. Continue chipping away at it until you feel the security you feel great and content with.

Great and extraordinary lovemaking doesn't mysteriously occur independently from anyone else. It requires exertion and investigation. On the off chance that you and your partner consented to be cozy and are encountering sexual movement together, at that point there is no compelling reason to fear from investigating each other's bodies. Take as much time as necessary to respect and contact the subtleties of your partner's body. Genital contact has a greater effect than the vast majority think. Watching your partner's body will develop your thankfulness for that person, just as stimulate you more. The person will likewise feel joy and uncommon, which is in every case great!

Discussing your intimacy with your partner may make you feel humiliated or senseless, yet it is something to genuinely consider on the off chance that you are not getting what you need and need behind those room entryways. In the event that you don't discuss, your dissatisfaction will just increment until you longer feel any craving to have intercourse with your partner. You two have a sense of safety enough to see each other bare, so having a discussion about it ought not to need to be an issue. Regardless of whether you are in general happy with your lovemaking schedules, discussing despite everything, it does great to your relationship since you will recognize each other's extraordinary lovemaking aptitudes, value one another, and move you nearer together.

Exercise consistently requires a decent warm so as to show signs of improvement results. The equivalent goes for having intercourse. You should never simply hop into it since it demonstrates the lower esteem you put on the close time you share with your partner. Of course, there are times you will need to be unconstrained and simply put it all on the line, however, and still, at the end of the day, you can't simply request it and take it. Add some sentimental fixings to your lovemaking course. Models would be, going out to your preferred sentimental café, viewing nightfall on the seashore, viewing a motion picture you both appreciate, giving each other an erotic massage, scrubbing down together, etc. Discover what works best for you!

Couples who have been as one for some time never again want to play with each other. They feel it is something individuals do when they are single and attempting to score with somebody. Being a tease is shockingly better when you are seeing someone. You both know one another and have a sense of safety; making you progressively agreeable to state whatever is at the forefront of your thoughts. So, feel free to play with your partner and bother that person into the room!

Orgasm Fulfillment

As indicated by Merriam Webster lexicon, climax the quick pleasurable arrival of neuromuscular pressures at the stature of sexual excitement that is generally joined by the discharge of semen in the male and by vaginal withdrawals in the female. The orgasm feels unfathomable and there is nothing amiss with staying with the strokes and contacts that you know carries you to the edge everything.

In any the same old thing, all the time wears out a person's soul. You wouldn't eat a similar three dinners consistently, nor would you wear a similar outfit again and again. Each peak can feel distinctive as far as power and term, contingent upon how and what some portion of your body is being stimulated, she includes. Other than giving a physical discharge, it's likewise a passionate one—enabling you to feel nearer to your partner or just de-worry following an intense day. A few sorts of climax centers around the vagina in particular; others enable you to feel an earth-convulsing force in spots you never thought of as erogenous zones. You deserve to discover the joy your body can involve.

Chapter 1: How To Introduce Couple Games Into Your Bedroom

Long-term relationships and residing in the same house bring loads of everyday habits into our lives, difficulties start to extinguish passion, and soon enough sex has the risk of becoming that same "Saturday habit". This happens frequently because daily matters and life complications dwell so much in our thoughts than romantic evenings together, as happens in the first few months of a candy-bouquet relationship period.

Unspoken discontent, unresolved problems or accumulated aggression - all this must not be in your family life, because they are followed by quarrels, resentment, a cold and insipid bed. Sexual games are a way to get rid of daily stress, get pleasure, support the sensuality and sexuality, and at the same time not offend each other, but rather ignite. Role-playing games in bed make it possible to transform into a character and act as you would never dare in everyday life. This transformation makes it possible not to be shy, not to select words and actions, because you both understand that this is only a game.

Role-playing in bed can solve some family problems. How does it work? Roles for the game can be very different, the

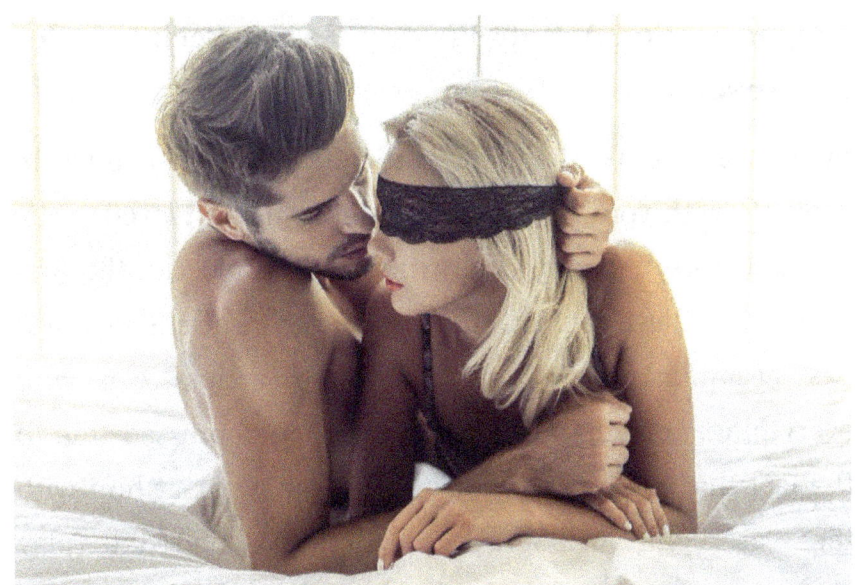

plot is much more important. For example, in each couple, one partner always dominates. In the role-playing game, you have the opportunity to switch places: if the husband takes decisions in everyday life, then become a strict teacher and punish him for his bad behavior. Also, a common problem in relationships, when we release the anger and discontent accumulated over the day on a partner, although a loved one is not to blame for your failures at work or other individual areas of life. So that problems outside the home do not be reflected in the relationship, transfer them to the game. If a man comes home after a heated debate with his boss, let him be the boss that night and to write you a few reprimands.

Preparing For A Role-Playing Game: Script, Rules And Inventory

First of all, think about the difficulties and innuendos in your life with your partner. If you have never played erotic games before, this approach will help you pick up the first roles and relieve tension in the plane of relations where it has accumulated. Incorrect roles or scripts can ruin everything. Imagine a man is constantly depressed due to the fact that his girlfriend has been you swear at him with the reason and without, and here he is offered to play mistress and her page-boy - the same situation that usually. Even if a man agrees, this game is unlikely to bring him pleasure, which, as in any sexual intercourse, should be mutual.

Try to carefully lead your partner to what worries him, to identify painful points, catch random phrases, but you should not talk about it openly, because you risk turning everything into a small home scandal, rather than a fun game. Next, select the roles that would enable you or your partner to "recoup." It will not be superfluous to learn about his fantasies, but absolutely everyone has them. So that the game does not come to a standstill or go in the wrong direction (for example, you should have been mistress, and then the man took the initiative again), write a simple, uncomplicated scenario. It is not necessary to think through all the dialogues to the smallest detail, but the general direction should be determined.

Sexy Outfits Play An Important Role In Erotic Games.

Another option to decide on the roles is to delve into yourself: think about what you would like to try, what erotic fantasies visit you, what kind of dress or atmosphere you like most.

The next stage is - outfits. Dressing up is a lot of fun. And understanding what kind of clothes can arouse your sexual desire can make this activity even more fun and enjoyable. Even the most ordinary objects can be filled with sexual vibration. Everything is simple here - either rummage through your own closet in search of suitable clothes (for example, you will definitely find something for the role of a teacher or boss) or look into a sex shop (not every house has a nurse's robe or a pilot's uniform). When you have figured out the costumes, think about what equipment may be needed so as not to run around the apartment in the middle of the game in search of a pointer, stethoscope or pipi aster - everything should be at hand

Mandatory Role-Playing Rules

- The game begins a few hours before the action. Send a thematic message to your partner (for example,

"Doctor, I have a headache, can I make an appointment with you tonight?") - at this moment you are already playing, so exclude the everyday messages "Buy bread". Similarly, you can throw a secret note to your partner, but you need to make sure that he will find it. It will be a shame if you put it in your trouser pocket, and he put on jeans.

- Do not start if you are not sure that you will reach the end. The worst thing is to tease each other with messages during the day and change your mind at the last moment. Such turns will not benefit your relationship.

- Do not change clothes and do not get ready in front of each other. You should meet for the first time already in full uniform and outfits, otherwise, the "magic" will not work.

- Play to the end. None of the partners in the middle of the game can take off the suit and get out of the role. Firstly, sex runs the risk of passing as usual, and not playing the psychological role for which, everything was started. Secondly, you can offend the efforts of a partner, which will only aggravate problems in the relationship.

- Improvise. If you initially did not have a ready-made

script, or it was not implemented, and the game slows down, do not freak out. The phrases "I don't know what's next," "Think of it yourself," "Maybe you can play along with me?" – they are a taboo! It's better to think in advance where the plot might go, and what to do in such cases. In any case, even if you found the problem of interpersonal communications during the game, do not concentrate on it, urgently turn your attention to any aspects that pleasantly excite you in this situation, move the focus to the exciting details, to immerse yourself in the game deeper and not lose your sexual mood. You can reflect and gently discuss all points for improvement afterward, in a more suitable atmosphere.

- Do not try to be a great actor. To read the monologues from Hamlet in front of the partner is completely unnecessary. Focus on the main goal of the game - quality sex. If you are playing not as George Clooney, believe me, the partner is unlikely to notice this and certainly will not criticize you.

- Do not go over the role of others. If the partner dominates in the scenario, do not drag the blanket over yourself. Similarly, if you dominate, - do not let the partner go over you, you will have to be tougher, but do not go too far - for inexperienced players, the line is rather thin. It's best to clarify the rules in advance.

- Do not undress ahead of time. If you threw off clothes from each other at the very beginning, the game already failed, because the very interesting stage of flirting was lost.

- It may sound corny, but some erotic games, especially with the use of BDSM toys, require to have "stop" words. The word should be simple, but atypical for the script. If you play, for example, in a clinic, then you should not choose a "dropper" with a stop word, it's better to choose something out of the ordinary, for example, a "bullfighter" - it's unlikely that you were going to discuss the bullfight in the script.

- It is preferably that you will be home alone at this time; the phones should be shut down.

- You should be as tactful as possible, sometimes even an innocent joke can bring down the whole mood, and then the partner in the future will completely refuse such entertainments.

- Don't think about anything extraneous, if at the height of the game a kitty instead of "murmur" suddenly says that tomorrow she needs to call on her mother, then this greatly disturbs the mood.

Chapter 2: Roleplaying Sex Games

One of the easiest and fun ways to overcome sexual inhibitions is role-playing. Sexual role play is a game that involves acting out sexual fantasies using different roles that may be completely unlike the individuals in real life. The intensity of the play depends on the participants. You can choose to role-play using makeshift props or go into elaborate preparations complete with scripts and matching costumes for each character in the play. However, you don't need to be an award-winning actor/actress or even have any prior experience in acting to enjoy sexual role play.

The Process

Bring Up Your Mutual Sexual Fantasies

Unless you want to take your partner by surprise and hope that they play along, it is usually better to brainstorm different ideas and scenarios with your partner. Come up with what you each think is agreeable. We all have sexual fantasies even if we don't actually want them to happen in reality. But these fantasies could be your guide to enjoying role-play with your partner. Perhaps you wish your masseur or masseuse would be a bit more daring and take things just a bit farther during your massage sessions, or you have always had an eye for one of your teachers back in college.

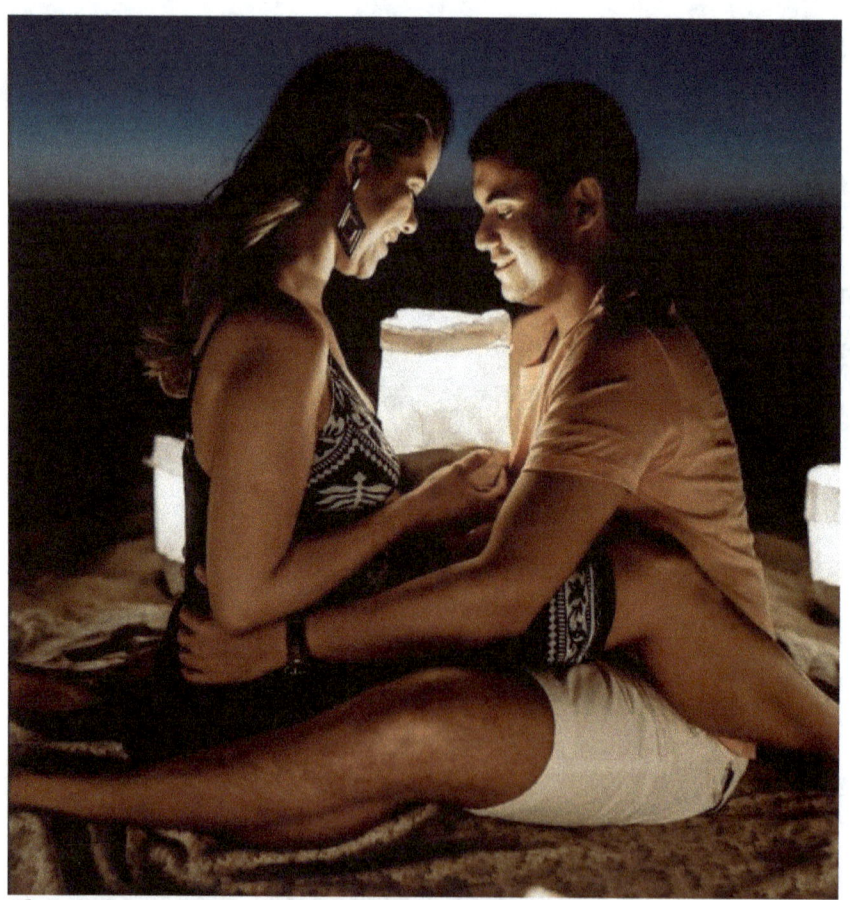

Share those fantasies with your partner and see which ones both of you can act out.

It is crucial to do this because one partner's idea of role-playing may be too strong or kinky for the other. But when you talk things out together, you will figure out what works for both of you. Anyway, it is a good idea to remain having an open mind and think of it all as mere fantasy and nothing more.

You can start with simple settings at first. Getting into too many details and imagination may be too daunting for you or your partner and defeat the goal of sexual role play. Start with something that can be done in a familiar setting such as your home or a nearby restaurant or bar. Select simple roles/characters and scenarios such as:

- A lonely businessman and the comforting sexy woman at a bar or restaurant.

- A pervert teacher and the naughty student in a class or the teacher's office.

- A nurse and her sick patient in a hospital bed.

- A house owner and his sexy maid in the living room or kitchen.

Dress the Part If You Wish

Go ahead and dress the part if it will help you to play the part more realistically. You can buy hats, wigs, and other costumes from costume shops, online, or adult shops. While costumes can add more excitement and fun to the whole idea of role-playing, they are not a requirement. Only get them if you think you really need them. Moreover, you may not have extra money to spend on costumes and props or you just want to keep things simple. Several roles require little to no costumes (a stranger at the bar, being on a blind date, and so on).

Make It Kinky If You Wish

Some sexual role-plays (such as officer and criminal, teacher and student, boss and secretary) are more about power and dominance. One partner (the dominant) gets to have their way with the other (the submissive). If you want to explore sexual dominance or kinkiness in a more relaxed and playful atmosphere assume the dominant/submissive roles using any character of your choice.

However, role-play is not all about power exchange. You can choose to skip any role that tends to portray the dominant/submissive attributes.

Start Slow

As always, it is best to start anything new with baby steps. It may feel too unreal, ridiculous, or just plain silly to get all dressed up and act like someone else. But you don't have to dress up to start with. Playing pretend may seem like a childish thing to do, but if you let go and play along for just a little while, you may discover that you are actually turned on by the idea of picking up a stranger at a bar, for example (even if you've known this "stranger" all your life).

Even if you totally buy the idea of sexual role play, it is wise to start slowly. You can begin by sending a raunchy text or sext detailing your sexual fantasy to your partner. This can be another form of foreplay. If you are a shy person, you can use this medium to open up communication on potentially awkward or embarrassing sexual subjects.

Let Your Character Use Dirty Words

There is no movie director here; it's just you and your partner. That is why you don't need to be uncomfortable if you get your first few lines completely wrong. Feel free to laugh about it if you fumble or make mistakes. No one is taking a score. Just let yourself ease into character and the words will flow naturally. You may or may not know how the fantasy will end. In any case, simply let your imagination guide you into what your character will say and say them without reservation. Even if you don't like profanity or filthy words, your character may like them. Permit your character to say what they need to say to make the game fun and exciting.

Sexual Roleplay Ideas

Here are a few sexual roleplay ideas to help stimulate your imagination and get the ball rolling. You are welcome to tweak them to suit you and create your own dirty dialogues along with it. You can use the dirty phrases in parenthesis as part of your sex dialogue.

1. Play the role of a firefighter who just rescued your partner and is rewarded with sex. (Dirty phrase: "You saved my life. The least I can do is to offer you my dick/pussy.")

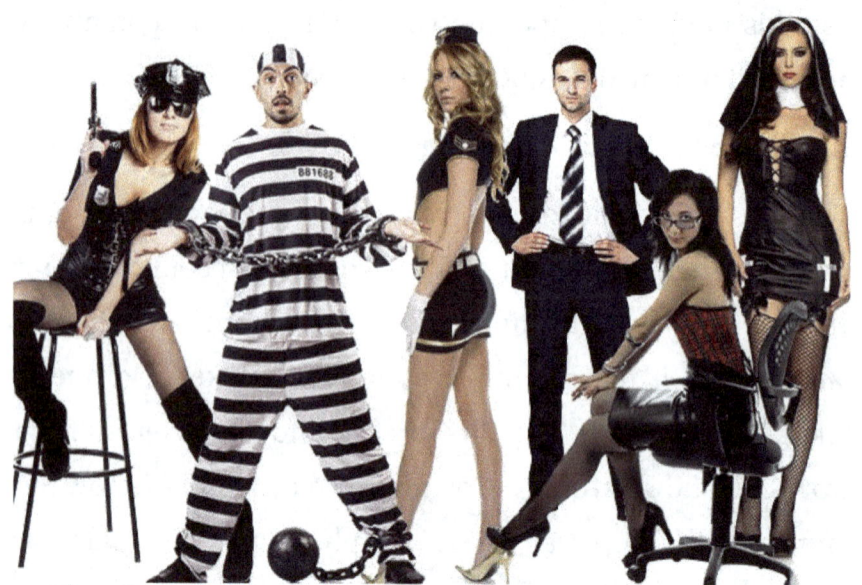

2. Play the role of a cop. Your partner is trying to get wriggle their way out of a speeding ticket. (Dirty phrase: "The only way to get out of this is to please me.")

3. Play the role of a prostitute who's just having sex for the cash. (Dirty phrase: "Show me the cash and I'll give you good pussy/cock.")

4. Pretend you came for a sleepover at your friend's and snuck out to have sex with your friend's sibling. (Dirty phrase: "Shhh... come have a taste of this cock/pussy before someone sees us.")

5. Pretend that you are a client getting a massage from your partner who is a masseur or masseuse and is willing to give you a happy ending. (Dirty phrase: "Could you go a bit lower... lower still, yeah... that's the spot.")

6. Pretend to knock on the wrong hotel room door but the stranger who opened up (your partner) invited you in any way. (Dirty phrase: "Never mind, I could use the company of someone as gorgeous as you are right now.")

7. Play the role of a landlord who's come to collect their rent, but your partner can't pay, so they end up paying in kind. (Dirty phrase: "I'm gonna fuck my money's worth out of you tonight.")

8. Play the role of a yoga instructor teaching your partner how to stretch and bend over. (Dirty phrase: "Nice and slow... that's it. Now bring that sexy ass of yours over here.")

9. Play the role of a boss who is about to have sex with his or her employee on the desk. (Dirty phrase: "I see you've been striping me naked with your eyes all day. It's time to turn this office into our sex haven!")

10. Both of you should assume the role of angry partners in a rough sex session.

11. Play the role of a tour guide with a strong accent. Let your partner listen to your dirty talk with a different accent.

12. Recreate the roles of your favorite porn stars from a porn scene or novel.

13. Play the role of a naughty maid trying to have quick sex with the house owner before the wife shows up. (Dirty

phrase: "I'll be in the kitchen... I've got no pants on. Hurry!")

14. Pretend to be a dance teacher and seduce your student (partner) through your movements. (Dirty phrase: "Place one foot ahead of the other and move your hips this way. Gosh! You look so sexy in that pose!")

15. Play the role of a hooker trying to get a one-night stand. (Dirty phrase: "I'm free for the whole night. Would you like to do something fun and sexy?")

16. Play the role of a pizza guy who gets a blow job in place of cash. (Dirty phrase: "I'm sorry I don't have any cash at home. But I'm sure we can figure out some other more interesting way to pay?")

17. Pretend is your first sex as husband and wife on your wedding night. (Dirty phrase: "I've been waiting for this moment all my life. I can't wait to finally be inside you / have you inside me!")

18. Play the role of an artist and paint your nude partner on a canvas. (Dirty phrase: "You have the curves of a god/goddess.")

19. Play the role of a shy virgin having sex for the very first time. (Dirty phrase: "Promise to be gentle with me tonight, would you?")

20. Play the role of an innocent person who is completely

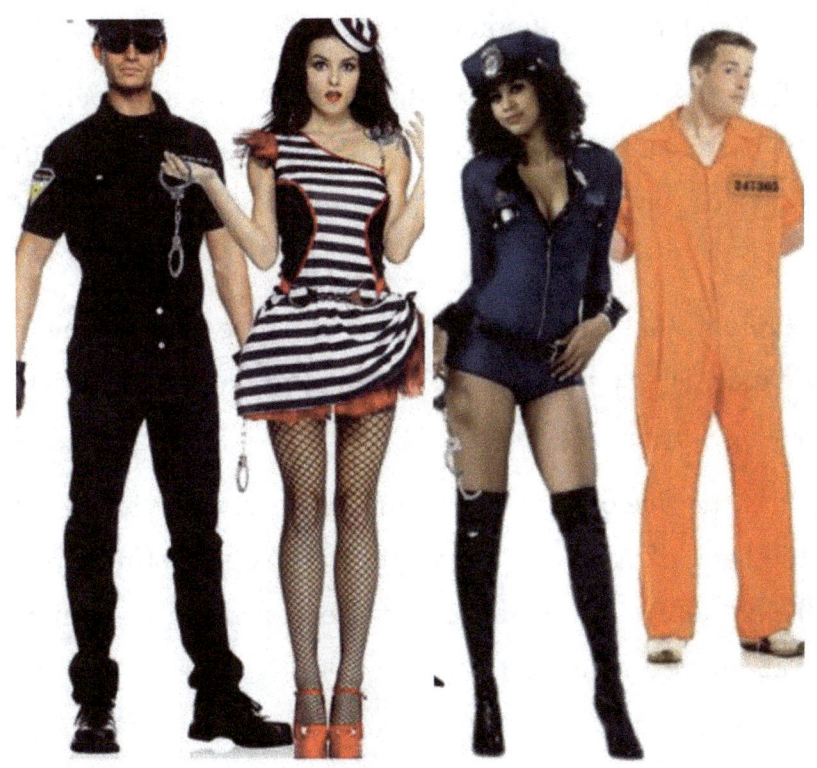

naïve about sex. Let your partner teach show you how to have sex. (Dirty phrase: "Is that what an erect penis/aroused vagina looks like? Oh... I see.")

21. Pretend you are a student who's trying to seduce their teacher for better grades. (Dirty phrase: "I might not be good at algebra, but I can tell from the way you look at me that you want to have a taste of me, don't you?")

22. Pretend that you are a hypnotist who has hypnotized your partner. Command them to do whatever you wish. (Dirty phrase: "You will suck my cock / eat my pussy when I

instruct you. Nod if you understand me.")

23. Play the role of a nurse and bathe your "sick" patient (your partner). (Dirty phrase: "If you would step out of your robe. Good boy/girl. Now relax let me take good care of you.")

24. Pretend that you are a striptease and give your partner a lap dance. (Dirty phrase: "Do you like it when I bend over and shake my ass like this?")

25. Play the role of a cab driver and have sex with your client in the back of your car. (Dirty phrase: "Your destination is still a bit far. I suggest we stop here for a while, grab a quick bite and have a quickie.")

Chapter 3: Classic Erotic Games

In this part, we will look at ways to spice up your sex life with some fun games and challenges you can play, of the erotic variety of course. Including sexy games and challenges will keep your relationship fun and flirtatious for a long time to come and these you can keep changing and introducing new ones to keep the experimentation alive. You may have played innocently flirtatious games in middle school like spin the bottle or 7 minutes in heaven. We're gonna use a common idea of fun and games but a much less innocent variety. These games are designed for you and your partner to have some sexy fun together. You can use this as foreplay or as fun in the evening. It doesn't have to progress to full-blown sex, but I assure you that you both will be heavily turned on after playing one of these that you will not be able to wait to get to penetration. Just try not to come too early on in the game!

Never Have I Ever

This game is a fun way to learn more about your partner's sexual history, but in turn, they will also learn about yours! Both of you will begin with five fingers up- these represent your lives. One of you goes first and says something they have never done, for example: "Never have I ever had a threesome". If your partner has done it, they have to put

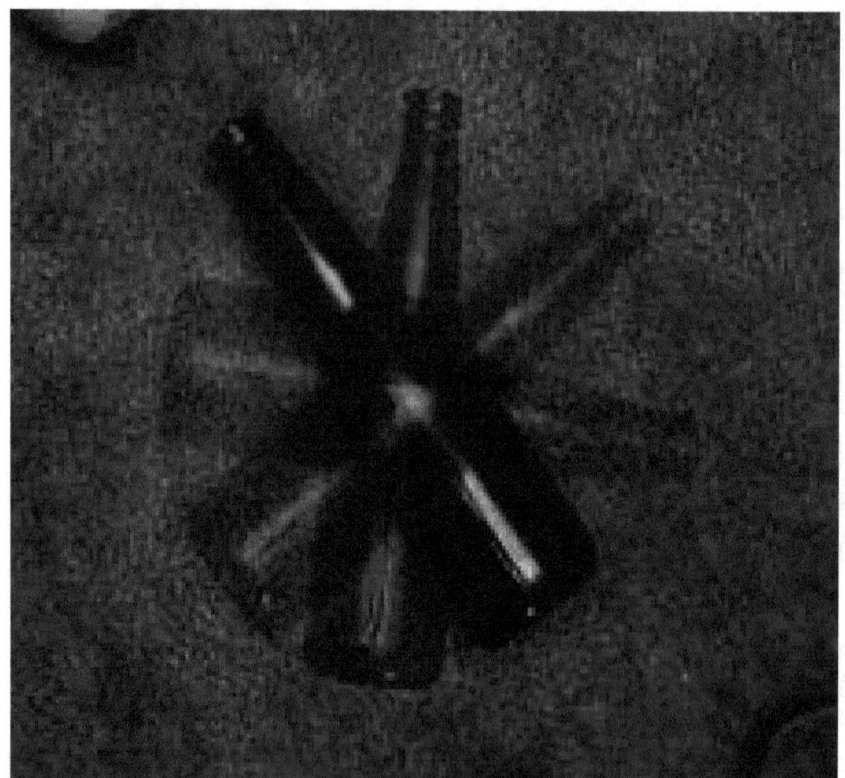

down one finger. You go back and forth like this and the first person to lose all of their lives loses the game! The loser will then have to give the winner something of their choosing. This game can also be played as a drinking game where, instead of lives using fingers, if the other person has done the thing you say they have to take a sip of their drink. If you play this way, it can go on for quite a while since there are no lives. To keep it fun and lighthearted, say things that you have not done, but that are not targeted at the other person such as "never have I ever been named John" if your partner is named John. Keep it fun and sexy by saying things related to dating, sex and all taboo topics you can think of. Play this game with the intention of getting to know your partner better and having them get to know you better as well.

Spin the Bottle

Traditional spin the bottle is done in a large group of people with each person being an option the bottle can land on. Everyone sits in a circle with the bottle lying on its side in the middle. You spin the bottle on its side and whoever the opening is facing when it stops spinning is the person that you have to kiss.

In this spin on spin the bottle, we are going to switch it up a little bit. You can play this game with anything you have, all you'll need is some type of bottle, some paper, and a pen. Think of the regular spin the bottle circle, with 6 or 8 people all sitting in a circle. Instead of people, we are going to have one challenge at each spot. At each spot, there will be a piece of paper with a challenge written on it, and whichever spot the bottleneck is facing after your spin

- Lick my nipples

- Give me a hickey

- Give me oral sex for 2 minutes

- Pick which position we will have sex in after this game

- Strip down to your underwear

- Give me a massage on a body part of my choosing for 2 minutes

- Give me a lap dance

- Take off my shirt using your teeth

- I will look for the craziest sex position I can find online and you attempt it with me

Ice/ Candle Challenge

For this game, you will need some small ice cubes and a small candle that has been lit for at least a few minutes. First, using the piece of ice, slowly rub it down your partner's chest between their nipples and down their stomachs. This will make their skin cool and numb. Then,

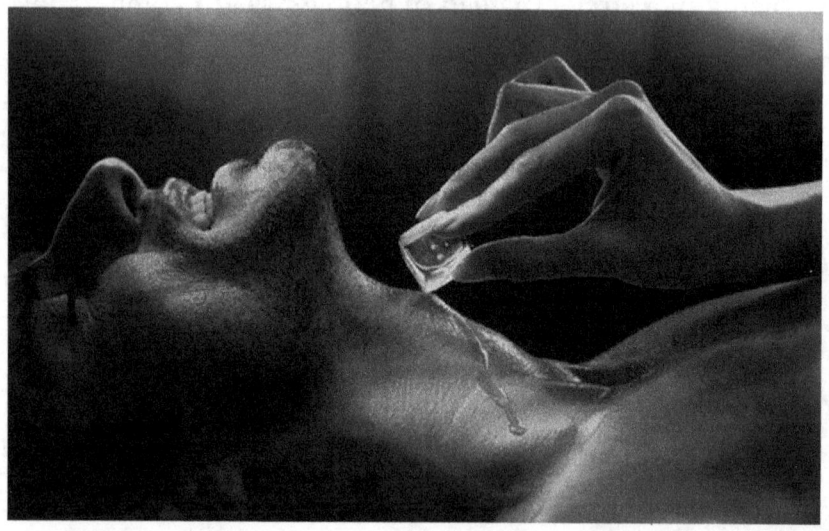

using the candle, carefully and slowly drip some wax on their chest and down their stomach, on the same spots that you rubbed the ice cube. This quick transition from cold to hot will make their skin tingle with sensitivity and when you touch them there their senses will be heightened. You can move to other spots on the body as well, like the back of the legs or the feet. Have fun with this as a little game to play during foreplay.

Whipped Cream/ Chocolate Challenge

Another, similar challenge to the Ice and Candle Challenge, is the Whipped Cream Challenge. Using either whipped cream or chocolate sauce, spread it down your partner's chest all the way to their belly button and down their pelvis, stopping just before their sensitive clitoris or the base of their penis. Slowly lick it off of them in the sexiest way possible. Once you have set the mood for a fun and sexy licking experience, you can get closer and closer to their genitals. A spot that would feel amazing for a man is if you put chocolate sauce on his testicles, and slowly licked it off of them, gently sucking every last drop off. Watching you do this will drive him crazy. Take turns doing this challenge and you can both clean off after with some steamy shower sex.

Truth or Dare

Play sexy Truth or Dare with your partner. Just like when

you were young, a game of Truth or Dare helps you get to know people in a funny and sometimes daring way. If you have no idea how it is played, I will explain the rules first! Each partner takes a turn asking the other person "Truth or Dare?" The person responds with their answer, and depending on which they choose, a truth- a question that they have to answer truthfully, or a dare- a challenge that they have to complete, is given to them. If they do not complete the dare or will not answer the truth question, they have to accept a pre-determined punishment. This punishment can be to take a shot (If you are playing a drinking version) or to give you a massage, anything you wish. Decide this punishment at the beginning of the game. As you play, you will make up truths or dares for your partner that get them to tell you or do things to you that are fun and sexy!

Below are some examples of truths or dares that you can give them:

Truths:

- Tell me your wildest sexual fantasy

- What did you think about/imagine/ watch last time you masturbated

- What is your favorite sexual memory

- What is something you have always wanted to try during sex?

- What is the naughtiest thing you have ever done?

Dares:

- Lick peanut butter off of somewhere on your body of your choosing ex. finger, chest

- Turn the lights off and try to turn the other person on using only sounds

- Do a striptease to a song of your choosing

- Make out with their belly button

- Demonstrate their favorite sex position with a pillow

- Give them a lap dance

- Give them a hickey

Pillow Fight

What's better than a good old naked pillow fight? Pillow fights are fun and flirty and will remind you of simpler days. Having an innocent pillow fight with the person you love will restore a sense of fun and light-heartedness in your life. Doing this pillow fight while naked will be even more fun than any pillow fight you've ever had. When you both get sweaty and horny from seeing your partner jumping around naked in front of you, take it down to the sheets and enjoy every inch of their glistening body.

Simon Says

Simon Says is another childhood game, but this time with a sexy twist. In this game, one person is the caller or Simon. This person can tell the other person to do something whenever they want just by saying "Simon says" before it. For example, they could say "Simon says, bring me a glass of wine." Then, a few minutes later while drinking their wine they could say "Simon says give me a foot rub." You can give the person a time limit to get everything they want out of it, say 5 or 10 minutes. You can play this game over the course of an evening while you do other things. If you want to fully focus on this game, you can take turns saying Simon Says, so each person has one turn as Simon and then it alternates. Start out easy and progress to sexier and sexier asks. Get creative with this game and make it as sexual as possible!

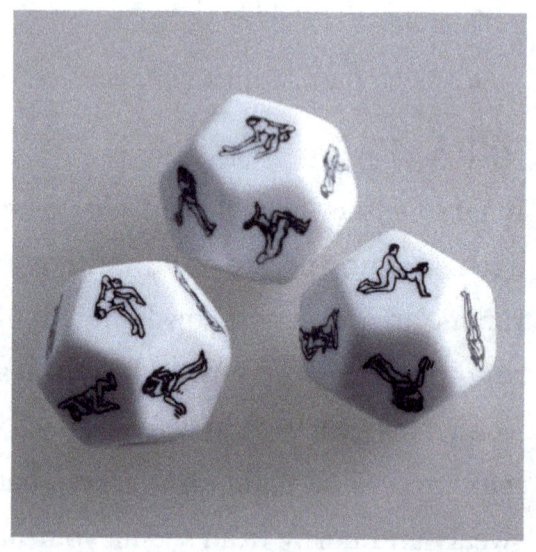

Sexy Dice Game

Write down 12 sexual acts that you want to do with your

partner, or acts that you want to have one person do for the other. These can be sexy, cute or funny. Write each one of them on a different piece of paper. Roll two dice together and add up the numbers you get. Whatever number you roll corresponds to the sex act written on that paper. The person that rolled the number will then have to perform the act to or with their partner. Take turns rolling the dice and keep performing the acts that you get.

These could be things like the following;

- Kiss my feet all over

- Suck on both of my nipples for 10 seconds each

- Give me a buttocks massage for 2 minutes

- Write "I love you" on my stomach with your tongue

- Massage a body part of my choosing

- Give me an orgasm using only your tongue

- Tell me your most secret sexual fantasy

Strip Trivia

Be certain that both of you and your partner are wearing the same amount of clothes first. Then, you are going to test your partner's knowledge of you by playing strip trivia! You will each take turns asking the other person something about you. These questions can be things like your favorite color, your mother's maiden name, your childhood home's house number- anything. If your partner's answer is incorrect, they have to take off an item of clothing. If they get the answer right, they get to put an item of clothing back on. If you want to make it harder, you can take out that second rule of being able to replace an item of clothing and can decide that if an item of clothing is taken off, it is gone for good. You better hope that you know your partner better than they know you or you'll end up naked first!

Chapter 4: Oral Sex Games

While some might think of oral sex as a form of foreplay, I've decided to cover it in a different part for a number of reasons.

For starters, there are several misconceptions about it. The very first thing to consider about oral sex is that you should feel comfortable with it, regardless if you are giving or receiving it. Make sure that you are doing it because you want to.

Secondly, oral sex is something that can go wrong very easily. There are good reasons why some people abstain from it. If you have thought of oral sex as something unpleasant, though, it is probably time to change your mindset or how you and your partner have been thinking about it.

We will focus on how to make of oral sex a more gratifying and pleasant experience for couples.

Basic Game Rules for Oral Sex

Before going deeper into this matter, let's talk about some ground rules. Frequently, when oral sex is practiced, we mainly concentrate on the person whose genitals are starring in the action. However, the one who gives oral does not have to be there only to please the other person. The giver shouldn't just lick and sip unscrupulously. In fact,

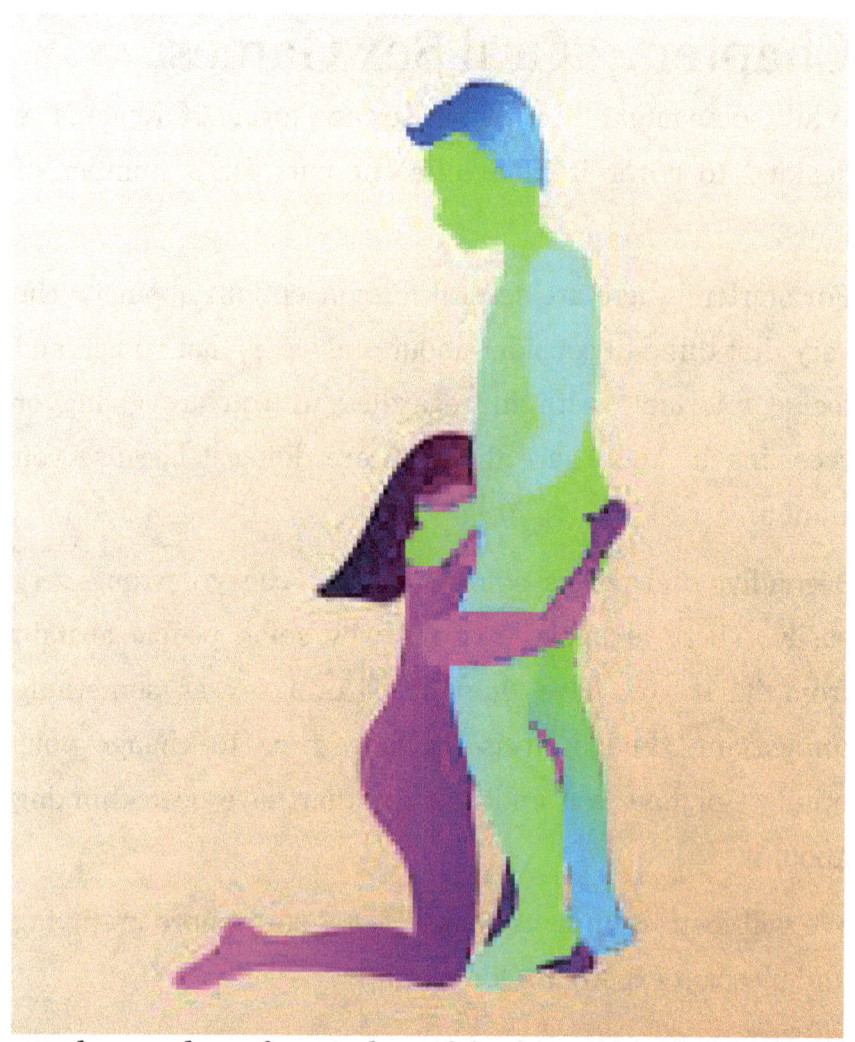

couples tend to forget that if both parties are enjoying themselves, the quality of sex increases respectively.

What is more, many women often complain that they feel arches, hurt their neck, or stay with their jaws dislocated after performing oral sex. I am not saying that a lot of men seem to be drilling into the vagina with their fingers rather than properly stimulating their partner's erogenous zones. What seems to be prevalent among both females and males is that they often forget that they can use their lips. Quite habitually, oral sex is performed only using tongues.

What you need to keep in mind is that oral sex is not just about "giving". Once you change that perspective, you will notice that it is not tiring and uncomfortable. When you start considering oral sex as a way to satisfy yourself and your partner, oral sex will be something that both of you are going to look forward to. In this sense, it is important to kick out some myths about fellatio.

First and foremost, a blowjob does not have to be a job for women to do. Men should also be willing to perform oral sex to their partners and do so with enthusiasm and on a regular basis. The more comfortable both parties are with this idea, the more enjoyable it will be with time.

It is evident that we all enjoy having a blowjob here and there. So, a first step forward is to be open to give without expecting to receive in return. Do not wait for your partner to ask you for oral sex. If you are up to the idea, be the one offering it to them and see how your partner reacts. If you like to be the one receiving, be honest with your significant other. While you might be shy about it, being sincere will help you to improve your relationship in a sexual and emotional sense.

With all of this mind, think about the following when having oral sex with your partner.

• When you are doing a blowjob, express yourself clearly. We all like to know that we are doing a good job. This can increase our desire to continue; it excites us and makes us feel sexy. We are behind the wheel and we want to know that we are going in the right direction. If you are receiving oral, do not be silent and congratulate your partner on the good work that they are doing. Let your partner know how much you are enjoying every single moment of it. On the contrary, if you are the giver, the possibilities of communicating might seem much more complicated.

However, be creative and let your partner know that you are also enjoying the moment. You can moan and produce noises with your saliva, tongue, or hands. Do not assume that your partner is having a good time just because they are the receiver. Read their gestures and moves instead. Tell your partner to guide you if needed as well. It is better to have such guidance instead of staying in the same spot without your partner feeling anything.

• Likewise, do not forget that comfort comes first. If the receiver is not in a comfortable position, it will take longer to reach the climax or even enjoy themselves. On the other hand, an uncomfortable posture will result in a much worse oral experience. The receiver or the giver may just want to finish as soon as possible.

If you are going to kneel down, use a good cushion so that your legs do not hurt at the end. If you choose to lie on the other person, try to find a posture in which the knees are not anchored or your neck is not unnecessarily contracted. Keep your hair pulled back so that it does not get into your mouth and change position whenever you need to take a break.

• Take care of your personal hygiene. Nothing is more disgusting than unkempt genitals when it comes to oral sex. Moreover, this is even a matter of health precaution. Although you may have never thought about it, approaching your partner's genitals right after eating some pork ribs is neither clean nor pleasant. A simple shower and toothbrush before having oral sex is everything you need. Why not even start having fun in the shower?

• Do not forget that you can use your mouth to further enhance oral sex. When practicing oral sex, you must remember that your fingers can help to give even more pleasure beyond the mouth. Use your hands to caress your partner's breasts, thighs, buttocks, or testicles. Women can use their fingers to stimulate their partner's prostate. Men, likewise, can address part of the vagina at the same time by using their fingers.

A full oral sex experience can't be complete if you do not use your hands to stimulate the erogenous zones as we have talked about before. Think of this as a dual game in which you are doubling the pleasure of your partner.

• Do not dismiss stimulating yourself at the same time. As I mentioned earlier, the fact that you are on the giving end does not mean that you shouldn't enjoy the occasion. While performing oral sex to your partner, masturbate yourself or use your other hand to rub your own erogenous zones.

Remember that self-excitement (when we are giving oral sex) is one of the most important aspects to fully enjoy the experience. In addition to simply thinking about it, let your partner know that you are also having a great time. There are so many non-verbal ways to do so, including looks, gestures, caresses, smiles, moans, etc. If you can do that, the experience will be much more enjoyable.

• If it makes things easier for both of you, depilate yourself. That also goes for men! Beyond the shame of getting a pubic hair out of your teeth hours after giving a blowjob or cunnilingus, it can be a little uncomfortable to the giver. You can drown yourself in so much pubic hair! You do not need to get rid of all the hair at once; a little trimming can make oral sex much easier for the giver.

• Let your partner know if you are just about to ejaculate. Despite what we see in porn, many women do not like to swallow the semen or pour it on their face. To make sure that the grand finale is as fun for her as the rest of the experience, it is recommended to bring a hand towards the penis before ejaculating and let her know that you are about to finish.

Although female ejaculation is not so common, a lot of men do not seem to know when their partners have reached an orgasm and would continue performing oral sex afterward. It is either because they cannot feel the contractions with the amount of saliva or they expect something quite spectacular to happen. Due to this reason, it is better to notify your partner when you are having an orgasm. It is not only for the sake of knowing that you have reached the climax but so that your partner can improvise to make the end even better.

• Be sure that your partner is also having a good time. Do not simply walk away after the orgasm. If you reached an orgasm first, make sure that your partner has their turn, too. Remember that a well-rounded oral sex experience should have both parties enjoying the moment.

Chapter 5: Fantastic Erotic Games

Strip Poker

The most fantastic of the erotic games that can be played in the bedroom is strip poker. Often, in fact, one goes in search of very complicated entertainment to stimulate desire, when perhaps the most effective one has been known for decades and can be practiced at any time.

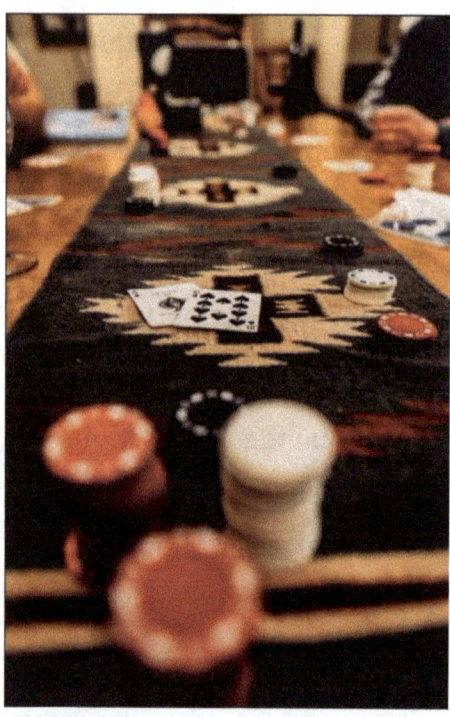

For those few who did not know it, strip poker is a very simple variation of poker in which garments are used instead of chips. So, when you "open" your hand or relaunch your bets, you will have to say you are willing to put your shirt, your bra or your underwear on the plate. And to give them the item in case you lose.

Therefore, a few materials are enough to play with it. Obviously you need poker cards and knowledge of the rules of the game, but above all an identical number of clothes. If the woman of the couple wears more clothes than the man, it is probable, he must put on something else to balance the bill.

Moreover, this is especially fun if you manage to create the right atmosphere. We suggest a suitable and intimate environment, such as that of the bedroom. The lights must be soft enough, so that you can see the fruit of your winnings but without making everything too loud.

Finally, when you lose a hand and are forced to take something off you, it would be good to improvise a small strip tease. Of course, it will be tastier to see the strip of her socks than his socks, but taking it with a certain irony, even the latter eventuality can be fun.

Erotic Dice

If you don't like card games, you can get rid of the playful aspect and go directly to penances. In specialized and online stores you will find, for example, dice that have been specially made to give you some interesting ideas. There are various types and they cost a few euros, but if you want you can also create them yourself. Just use, for example, traditional dice and a conversion table (1 corresponds to a penance, 2 to another and so on).

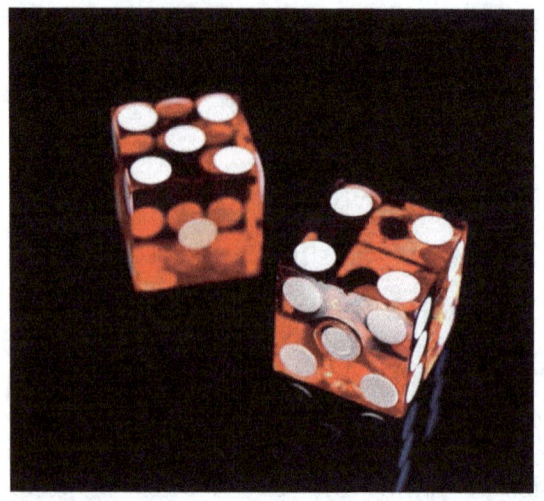

What can be found, however, in the various faces of these dice? For example, in one there can be actions and in the other the parts of the body. To be more concrete, in the first verbs such as "kiss", "suck", "pinch", "touch", "blow" or "lick" and in the second areas such as "chest", "lips", "ears", " neck "," sit "," navel "(or even worse, if you want).

Other dice, however, provide suggestions on sexual positions, like Kamasutra. They are often dice with 8, 10 or 12 faces with real explanatory drawings on the various sides. Rolling the dice, therefore, can force you to try things that have never been experienced before.

Monogamy

This is the first real erotic box game ever made. It is called Monogamy, it is produced by the British Creative Conceptions and is easily found in online stores. The game offers a game board with a circular path to be used by your pawn, and as you end up on the various squares you run into different cards. These cards - 100 for him and 100 for her -

each present 3 questions, with 3 different game levels. In addition there are also 50 fantasy cards.

The questions in particular allow us to investigate the couple's alchemy, and prove to be spot on both for the partners who have been together for a long time, and for the novices. In part, these are questions that investigate the other's mind, in part they suggest moving to action instead.

Erotic Twister

Monogamy is a game that must be purchased, and that must somehow wait for you to get home. If, however, it comes to your mind at the last moment, when it is already evening, to try an erotic game, you can orient yourself on a different solution. Use a classic box game, changing the rules.

This can be done with all games, perhaps with specific penances. Let's say that in Monopoly you don't have the money to pay when you pass over Victory Park: maybe your partner can give you a discount in exchange for some caresses.

However, there is also a game that already in its basic version is very suitable for an erotic evening: Twister. Remember it? It is that game in which a carpet with colored circles is placed on the ground, and then, by turning a small arrow on a dial, you understand where you need to put your hand or foot.

Obviously, when we play in many we end up meeting in improbable and improper poses. But in two poses they can also become subtly erotic. If the normal Twister is not enough for you, you can change the rules. Maybe placing a colored circle also on some sensitive areas of the body ("right hand on green buttock").

Tickling

In some areas of the world, in fact, this ancient practice has come back into fashion with the aim of preparing the couple for sexual intercourse. Tickling, in fact, allows you to create the right intimacy between partners and to touch in parts of the body that are not immediately sexual, but nonetheless erogenous.

You need not to use your fingers, but you can use other tools. For example, a feather passed on the neck (maybe behind) or on the back can have a particularly exciting effect. Some films then taught us the usefulness of using ice cubes, silk ribbons or even hair to caress our partner.

In this case, the important thing is to explore the other's body and find out which are the most receptive and sensitive points, in order to stimulate them adequately. Furthermore, the ideal would be to postpone the passage "to the facts" as much as possible, in order to enjoy this long but vibrant wait.

Lust

We told you about Monogamy, the perfect box game for couples. Well, that's not the only one you can use if you want to liven up an evening. Another available on the market is called Lust, and it is no coincidence that it is presented as a "Passion Play", a game of passion.

The game involves two players, who, through cards or specific moves, arrive at the end of a game by getting the suggestion of some sexual positions to explore. There are many combinations, more than 30,000, so that every time you can venture into an ever new experience.

Erotic Heart

Erotic Heart is also based on more or less the same principles, another game for couples that is actually marketed under various different names depending on the importer. However, its name is due to the fact that it is presented, right from the box, in a heart-shaped container.

Inside there are several rolled up notes, which the partners can fish one at a time. In each one is indicated a penance, but a very sweet penance, since it has an erotic nature that will surely be appreciated by the companion or companion.

Soft Bondage

There are also easier games to put into practice, for which there is no need to spend money or go to some shop. For example, bondage, practiced for a very long time even with very simple objects, such as ribbons or handkerchiefs (or even handcuffs and ropes, when you want to do things big).

Well, the game can be nice, especially if done in an undemanding way. In fact, soft bondage does not involve dangerous bonds, but only a few small games with laces and ribbons, preferably made of silk, in which to pretend and simulate even a little.

Smeared Food

Have you seen 9 1/2 weeks? The scene in which Mickey Rourke passes an ice cube over Kim Basinger's body is famous in that film. It is a very erotic scene, which at the time many tried to replicate even in the closet of their bedroom.

You don't have to use ice, actually. Indeed, with other elements - and in particular with food - the experience can be even more intriguing. Think for example of whipped cream, or strawberries, which are also aphrodisiac. In short, even here the fantasy is the master.

Erotic Apps

If your imagination doesn't really help to invent new sex games, you can resort to some erotic apps to install on your smartphone. For example, there is Planet Pron, a wide selection of videos and free images to whet your imagination, while for couple's sex games you can choose between Ultimate Sex Games for Couples for iPhone and The Foreplay Game for Android. If you want to try tantric sex instead, there is a Tantric Sex Deck. The important thing is that the apps are helpful for experimenting. The phone must not become an annoying third party! Unless you decide to use it for sexting: if a couple is forced to stay away, they can still carve out a spicy moment. In fact, at a distance you can exchange sexy images, perhaps through an app that does not leave a mark like Snapchat, and messages with a high erotic content. The only precaution is to always be attentive to privacy, and to do sexting only with a person you trust, in order to avoid unpleasant inconveniences such as the diffusion of photos and screenshots of the chats.

Chapter 6: Playing with Sex Questions

Romantic Revelations

When you're in a relaxed state before or after making love, softly caress your lover and entice them to reveal their romantic desires. Communicate pleasures that each of you wish to experience. Explore each other's special cravings that would make life that much more enjoyable. Discover each other's fantasies and discuss ways that they can be fulfilled.

1. Everyone has secret sexual desires that they believe are too sensitive, shocking or weird to reveal even to their partner. How can I make you feel more comfortable sharing our secret desires so we can both satisfy them together?

2. Some people think sexual fantasies should stay secret while others believe that it can be fun to reveal them and even turn them into reality. How do you feel about exploring and sharing our sexual fantasies?

3. What aspect of our lovemaking do you like the best? What is your favorite erotic memory of our time together?

4. How important is foreplay to you for great sex? What

makes for good foreplay?

5. If you were given the chance to "see" all the sexual thoughts, dreams and fantasies of just one person, whose mind would you want to read?

6. What is the "strangest" fantasy you enjoy and will admit to, but would never or could not actually do in real life?

7. How kinky or sexually adventurous do you feel:

You are?

I am?

We could be?

8. How curious about sex were you as a kid? What are the things you did to satisfy your curiosity?

Fabulous Foreplay

Use your creativity to engage your lover in a complete sensual experience that exhilarates their entire body and mind. Provide a feast for all five senses. Allow time to savor an entire range of sensory delights. When you make love next, strive to make foreplay absolutely fabulous.

9. How do you think we can make foreplay more fun? How would you most like to spice up our foreplay?

10. How do you feel about experimenting with creative new foreplay techniques? What new types of foreplay

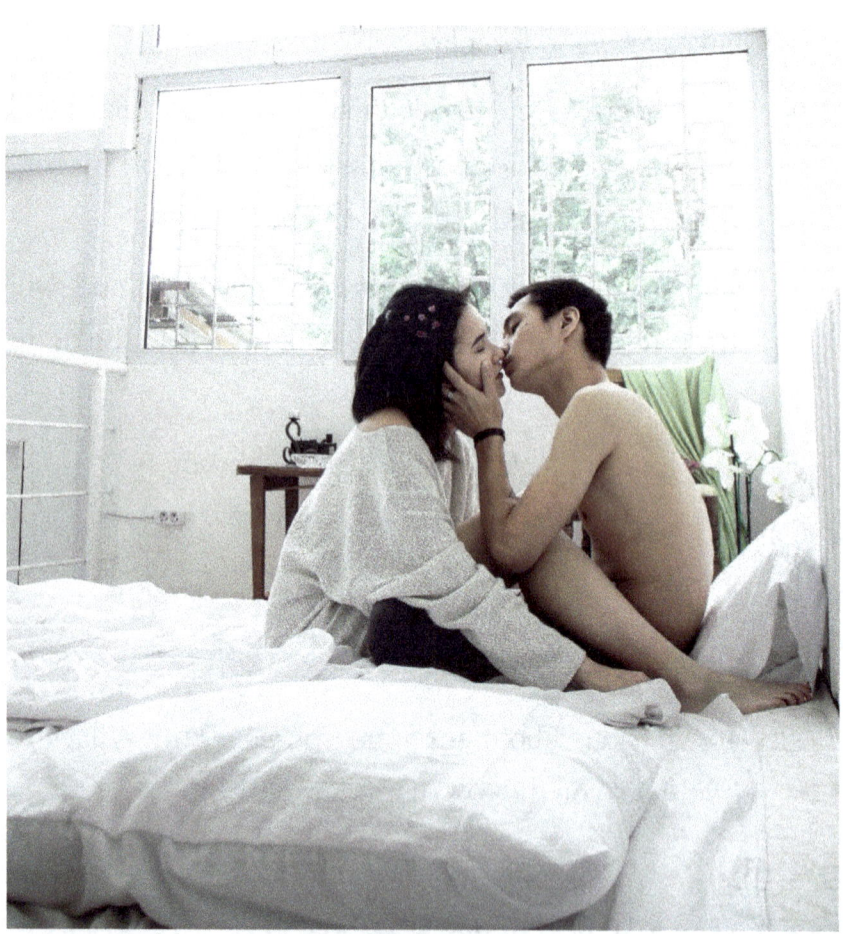

would you enjoy trying?

11. How do you feel about being blindfolded while I surprise you with pleasure? What types of foreplay techniques have you experienced while blindfolded?

12. How do you feel about watching porn together as foreplay?

13. Suppose we were making a penis mold that takes a while to set. How long do you think "we" could

maintain an erection and what types of stimulation do you think would be required to keep it hard?

14. Do you prefer to be spontaneous in what we do as foreplay or plan it out? In what ways do you like to mix up your foreplay moves?

15. What is your favorite foreplay technique that?

You use to pleasure me?

I use to pleasure you?

16. If we were to play out a modern day fantasy or role playing scenario, would you rather be:

Doctor or patient?

Escort or client?

Executive or assistant?

Cop or criminal?

Photographer or model?

Kiss Connection

The way a person kisses is a good indicator of how they make love. Improve your kissing style and range of techniques and you will inevitably improve your skill as a sensual lover. Even in established relationships, never take kissing for granted. Learn to kiss well and practice often. Combine different types of kisses in erotic patterns of sensual delight. Connect with your lover through the art of kissing.

17. How important is kissing to you? How can someone learn to be a better kisser?

18. In what ways do you feel we can improve the way we kiss each other? How can I improve the way I kiss you?

19. Where do you most like to be kissed other than on the lips?

20. What color lipstick do you think is most kissable? What color of lipstick do you think is the most erotic for oral sex?

21. Would you rather redo or relive the first romantic kiss you ever had? How do you think we can recreate the exciting sexual curiosity of our first make out sessions?

22. Have you ever had or given someone:

An electric kiss?

An upside down kiss?

A vampire kiss or hickey?

A snowball kiss?

23. How did you first learn to kiss? What else do you feel

we could learn about kissing?

24. What makes for a great kiss? What styles of kissing do you enjoy most?

Erogenous Exploration

With your lips and tongue, explore your lover's entire body. Resist the urge to concentrate on areas you already know. Map out new territory. Add some warm and cool breaths to further stimulate sensitive areas you discover.

25. What do you think are my most sensitive erogenous zones? Which part of my body do you most enjoy stimulating?

26. During foreplay, which of your erogenous zones or parts of your body would you like me to:

Touch and caress more?

Kiss and lick more?

Rub and massage more?

Stay away from?

27. With someone of the same sex, how would you feel about:

French kissing?

Performing a handjob?

Receiving a handjob?

Receiving oral sex?

Performing oral sex?

Having sex together?

28. How many different types of nipple stimulation can you think of? What forms of nipple stimulation do you enjoy most?

29. What household items can you imagine using to pleasure each other? What would we do with them?

30. What is the most imaginative foreplay technique you have ever experienced or heard of?

31. How would you most like to tease and tantalize me during our sex play?

32. In what ways do you think we can make our sex play more creative and erotically adventurous?

Luscious Lips

Use your lips to arouse your lover in ways they least expect or longingly desire. Explore their body for hidden erogenous zones or revel in a sensuous kiss. Keep your lips soft for all occasions.

33. What is your best tip or technique for performing great oral sex on:

A man?

A woman?

34. If I was naked and pretended to be a statue standing perfectly still, what would you do with just your tongue to make me move?

35. How do you feel about kissing after receiving oral sex?

36. What color would you associate with the word:

Love?

Sensual?

Sexy?

Passion?

Luscious?

Delicious?

Nasty?

Kinky?

37. How often would you prefer me to perform oral sex for you as:

Foreplay?

Your climax?

38. How do you feel about role reversal and gender play? What kinds of scenarios can you imagine us role

playing?

39. What is one foreplay technique you would like to try that we have not done yet? What is one sexual activity you would like to try that we have never done before?

40. If we were both sentenced to house arrest together for 6 months with no other responsibilities, what kinds of things do you think we would order online to make sure our sex play never got boring?

A Loving Touch

Use your fingers as delicate instruments of pleasure. Lovingly touch and stroke your lover's entire body. Sensitize their skin as you slowly explore for new erogenous zones. Take your time teasing and tantalizing until their genitals tingle with desire.

41. In your opinion, how is having sex different from making love?

42. What is your best foreplay tip if you were giving advice to:

A woman?

A man?

A lesbian?

A gay guy?

43. Are there any foreplay habits or routines that we have

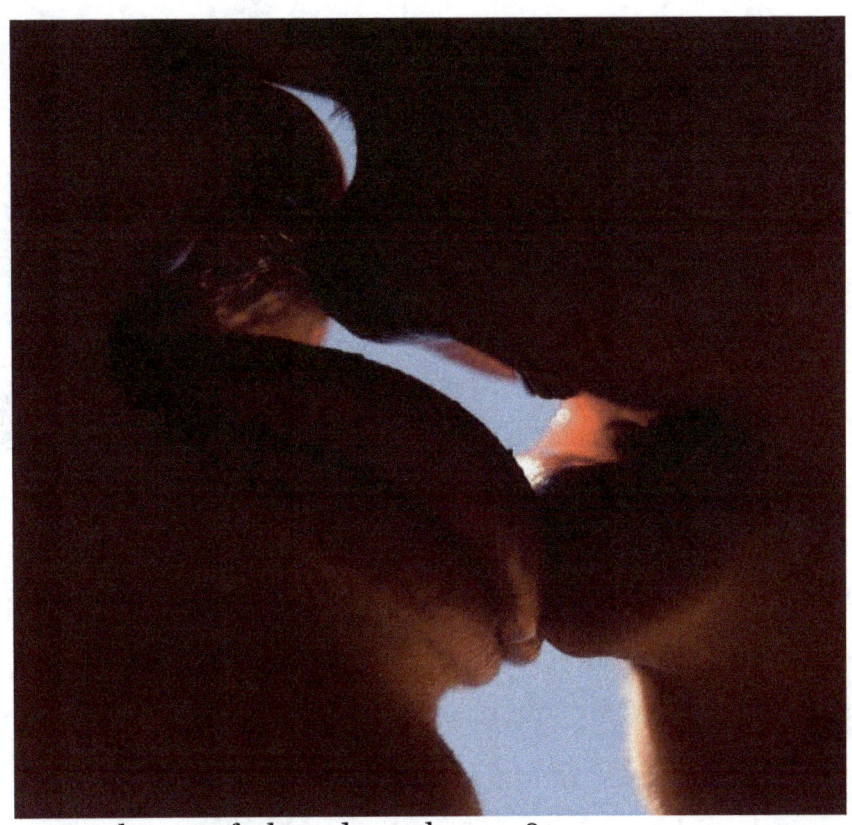

that you feel need a make over?

44. What sex toys do you have that you want me to use with you during our sex play?

45. Have you ever been involved in a threesome or more-some? If we were going to have another person or couple join us, who would you want to get together with and how would you imagine us doing it?

46. If we were to receive a prize for the most amazing sex scene, what would we have been doing together?

47. Think of a love story we've both seen together recently that had a happy ending. If you had to "finish" the movie with a sex scene, in what setting would the scene take place and what would the characters be doing?

Library of Love

Making love can be an art form when you fine tune your skills. Becoming a master of intimacy requires lots of practice combined with knowledge and a desire to learn. Invest in a private library of love. Learn creative techniques beyond your imagination. Discover ideas for new fantasies. Gain confidence as you discover the joy of learning. Buy a new book of love for your collection today.

48. What types of things do you do to improve your knowledge about sex?

49. What is your favorite type of erotic reading material?

50. In a fantasy or role playing scenario set in ancient times, would you rather be the:

Priest or worshiper?

Knight or the one rescued?

Barbarian or missionary?

Witch or inquisitor?

Traveler or native?

51. If we were to write an erotic story together, what would it be about?

52. What forms of sex education did you receive and how are you continuing to learn more?

53. If you had started a sexual scrapbook or memory box when you were a teenager, what kinds of things would you have put in it?

54. When it comes to playful activities that we can enjoy together:

Where do you get your sex play ideas?

Where is the best place to find creative ideas?

How can we come up with new ideas to try?

55. If you could go back in time to take photos or videos of your sexual history, what key events in your love life would you want to record?

56. Are there any foreplay skills you feel we need to learn or relearn?

Control of the Zone

When you master the erogenous zones of your lover, you will control awesome powers of pleasure. Wielding these powers to stimulate your lover with wonderfully subtle or intense sensations is a joy in itself. Watching them squirm in ecstasy as you control every nuance of their pleasure is extremely arousing. Take time to learn: explore and experiment, tease and test, seduce and study.

57. What are your most ticklish erogenous zones?

58. For mysterious reasons you wake up with a mixture of gender traits. Which mixture would you rather have?

A: Feminine features including breasts but with a penis and testicles

B: Masculine features but with a vagina and clitoris

59. Suppose you magically switched gender one night but kept all your existing personality traits. If you knew this was permanent, would you want to switch to an opposite sex partner (your previous sex) or "turn" gay?

60. What's the strangest thing you've done or thought about to avoid a premature ejaculation?

61. Would you ever consider timing ourselves to determine the fastest time to:

Strip and get into position?

Have a quickie?

Get an erection?

Perform oral sex?

Finish a hand job?

Have a G-spot orgasm?

Masturbate to orgasm?

Get into ten sex positions?

62. Have you ever gone sex toy shopping with a lover? While there, have you ever:

Squeezed a realistic dildo (texture & shape)?

Fingered a fake pussy to see what it feels like?

Tested a vibrator intensity on your nose?

Imagined fitting in the largest dildo they had?

Considered a sex doll for a pretend threesome?

Bought more than one sex toy at one time?

Chapter 7: Challenge Sex Games

What exactly is a challenge sex game?

It's where you are trying to accomplish a task during sex. It's usually going to be a task that involves some effort and focus, so it's challenging to complete both the task and a satisfying sex session. However, that doesn't mean we can't try and have fun in the process.

After all, it's through challenges and pushing ourselves to our limits that we find what we are capable of, and what we truly like. Above all else, it's just fun to try to turn sex into a game for you to conquer. As we all know, it's easy to get addicted to games that we haven't conquered yet, so these sex games may encourage you to have sex more frequently as well.

These aren't necessarily during foreplay or intercourse, they can be done and applied whenever you want to liven things up.

Lava Monster

Remember when you were a child and you played on the swings, there was a game where you had to stay off the gravel or tanbark? It consisted of you swinging from bar to bar, and making jumps from one area to the concrete and back.

Now, imagine that combined with sex. The floor (carpet, rug, wood, whatever you wish to define it as) has suddenly turned into steaming hot lava, and you can't touch it! You can have sex anywhere but the floor, but your task is to move from one room to the next.

You can take a maximum of three steps on the floor at a time, at which point you had better hop up on a table, counter, or chair and start having sex again. You only get three steps in between sex as well.

The more creative you get, the more fun this is. Start in the kitchen and work your way to your bed with only a couple of chairs and a rug to help you. How about figuring out positions that can work while one of you is standing, and the other is awkwardly twisted, trying to stay balanced? Or even walking through the house and stripping your clothes off, then having to follow that trail of clothing back to the bedroom without touching the floor underneath?

Remember, you can use more than just furniture. You can even, in desperation, grab a magazine or blanket from nearby and throw it on the floor to use. Be resourceful and have fun. It's best to start moving from just one room to another, and with plenty of objects in between. When you're ready for a bigger challenge, you can move across the house and back, taking different routes, using objects that only allow for one person to be stable at a time.

One Finger

This might be a challenge for some, and it might be extremely easy for others! The task here is to make your partner orgasm with just one finger. You take turns, and the one who can accomplish this the fastest wins. You can use other props, such as pornography, but your physical contact must be limited to one finger.

Men can finger, rub, and penetrate. You might think that the man has a distinct advantage in this because it's easier to focus on a clitoris as opposed to a penis with one finger.

That might be true, but there are plenty of ways women can stimulate a penis with one finger. Just focus on the crown of the penis, or if your fingers are long enough, wrap it around for a one-finger handjob. If it continues to be too unbalanced, simply move the goalposts, where victory for the man means two orgasms, and victory for a woman means only one orgasm.

This will again force you to be creative and resourceful and truly think, "How can I make an orgasm happen within these boundaries?" After all, necessity is the mother of invention, and you just might be inventing some unorthodox ways to create mutual pleasure.

Chase That Feeling

This sex game is a game of nostalgia and trying to recapture previous emotional and physical highs.

Each partner is going to think about the best sex they've ever had as a couple – with that specific partner. Then, you will think back to all of the circumstances surrounding it – what, where, when, why, how. Try to recall as much detail as possible about it, even if you fill in gaps with guesses.

You and your partner's best sex moments may not match, but that's okay. That just means you will take turns.

After you have filled in all the details about that moment, you will try to reproduce that sexual encounter as closely as possible with what you've taken note of.

If it was on the beach and you're far from the beach, use some sunscreen, put on ocean sounds, and sit on a towel on the ground. It if was in your car, drive your car to a dark alley (or maybe just your backyard) and do the deed there, playing the same music and wearing the same clothes. If it was in your bed after a long date, visit that same restaurant and order the same dishes before going home to do the dirty.

Just try to get the setting as similar as possible. This turns this game into a fun planning event for you two as well, because it will make you work together to build the scene.

As for the actual sex itself, try to emulate that too! Who made the first move, what happened, what positions you were in, and how penetration was first made. You can try to emulate the positions you used, and how and where you orgasmed as well, if you remember that. Did they do anything special that turned you on or surprised you? Did you cuddle afterwards and gear up for round two or did you have to hide from your partner's parents?

You are chasing an old memory, but simultaneously creating a new one, and perhaps even improving on it.

Name It

This sex game will test your sense of intuition.

Both of you will be naked. One partner will be blindfolded, and the other will be in charge of the game. The partner in charge will pleasure the blindfolded partner with an object for up to sixty seconds, and the receiver has three attempts to guess what the object is.

If the receiver is correct within those three attempts, then they are rewarded with whatever they want for sixty seconds. If they are wrong, however, they must change roles and blindfold the other partner. It will be more fun if you get creative and don't use sex toys. Instead, you can use household objects, food, clothing, unconventional parts of your body, or even sports equipment. You are only limited by your creativity what you can use to pleasure your partner!

Keep Rhythm

Music during sex is almost always a plus to set the mood and make it feel like you are in a world of your own.

This game takes it to the next level by requiring you to have sex to the beat of the song that is playing. To do this most effectively, look up a playlist on YouTube that changes songs or beats every sixty seconds. You can also set your normal music playlist to shuffle if that's easier for you. Just make sure that the songs played after one another are random and different in speed and rhythm.

Start this playlist when you begin foreplay, but you should really start paying attention when you start intercourse. Keep the beat of the music, stay in rhythm, and adapt when the song changes every minute. This will give you plenty of variety to play with, and make sure that the male and female have equal time on top, because the partner on top is essentially who controls the rhythm.

It would probably be worth your time to build a playlist of 60-second snippets ahead of time, just to ensure that the songs are of very different rhythms and speeds. For example, songs from salsa, techno, tango, and country are all very different and will make you move in a very different way. At the very least, you might discover new music that you like.

Staring Contest

This is a game you probably played as a child or with your cat, but it takes on a whole new meaning here.

This is mostly for use during intercourse. In this game, you and your partner will only have sex in positions where you can maintain eye contact. Missionary, cowgirl, side, whatever variations you wish to swivel into. Do your best to maintain eye contact the whole time, and don't break it unless you have to.

The first partner to look away or break eye contact loses a point. This game operates on a points system where the partner who has the higher score (whoever breaks eye contact the least) gets to choose a reward.

The staring contest sex game is great for a couple of reasons. First, it makes you feel more connected as a couple. That's what sustained eye contact can do, and it can make you feel like you can feel their soul, as well as their body. You may notice this session turns out to be more intense than normal for this very reason. Second, this becomes more difficult the closer we get to orgasm – we feel the need to look away or close our eyes. That adds a fun wrinkle, and puts you both on an even playing field!

Public Groping

We all have a little bit of an exhibitionist in us.

This game works by trying to touch your partner sexually as many times as possible in public.

The scoring system is as follows:

Grope penis/vagina over clothes: 1 point

Grope penis/vagina under clothes: 2 points

Grope penis/vagina over clothes for 5 seconds: 3 points

Grope penis/vagina under clothes for 5 seconds: 4 points

Oral under clothes (must be at least 3 seconds long): 6 points

You can see what you might want to prioritize if you want to maximize points! If you are caught, meaning a member of the public sees what you are doing, then you don't get the points. You can feel free to add different levels if the above is too daring or too tame for you.

Set the boundaries of this game to be an entire day, a trip to the mall, an errand, or out to lunch. Just make sure to agree on it beforehand so you don't end up fondling your partner in front of their parents.

Here's where it gets better: even though you are competing, you can both wear clothing that makes this easier for both of you. Skirts without underwear, elastic waistlines, short shorts, large baggy shirts, huge purses, big hats, and so on. If that feels too risky still, you can even alter your clothes to make it easier, such as cutting holes near the crotch or in pockets or pants so your partner can grope you in secret.

It will also help to think about specific locations where you can do this, such as photo booths, cars, dark corners, public restrooms, behind buildings, dressing rooms, and so on.

Public Groping can start as innocent fun, but can turn super hot and build incredible sexual tension, forcing you to race home unexpectedly from the gym because you are too aroused. Errands never looked so good!

Chapter 8: Games with Sex Toys

Hot and Dirty Scrabble

What You Need:

Get a Scrabble game and set it up on a cozy spot with several sex toys of your choice.

Both of you must start to scrabble with clothes on. List and agree on what will be the sexual favor or reward of the winner.

How to Play

The goal of Hot and Dirty Scrabble is to form words that express desire, lust and love for your loved one. Try to think of words that can arouse and make them horny for lovemaking. Based on the words you formed, get each other stripping and performing foreplay activities. The one who can come up with the highest score of a word will be the winner and be the one to receive the reward you set earlier Play the usual way you do with regular scrabble but with the following additional rules:

• For this version, terms that are slang are accepted as long as it is related to sex.

• If words are sexy and triggering, Multi-word combinations can be used (without spaces) (e.g., glass dildo, butt plug lick my)

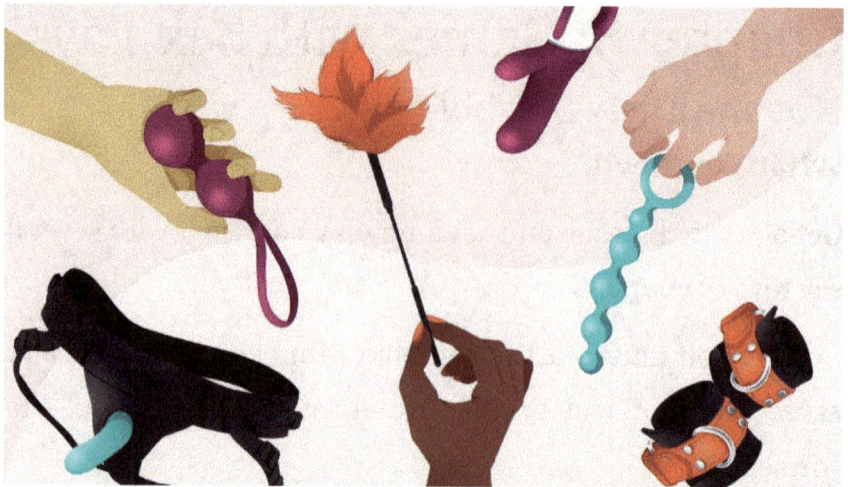

• Only one piece of clothing per turn can be removed for stripping.

• double or triple time will be given for sexy words placed on bonus squares Here are some words you can form to set off arousal.

• Shirt: I'll unbutton your shirt slowly.

• Flavor: Let me taste the flavor of this strawberry syrup when I lick and suck your breast

• Glass: Pleasure yourself with a glass dildo while I watch you.

• Black: Open your legs so I can please you with this black vibrator

• Paint: Use a clean brush to put lube around the clitoris and nipples

The Extension

What You Need:

For this game, an extender is used on the male partner. It is a shaft made to fit over his penis to create extra length and possibly girth. This can be done at home or perhaps a hotel

How to Play:

When the male partner uses this, he could be thought of as a new or different person to the female partner. Perhaps the two partners could simulate an affair, the female character is having. This could even lead to staying in a hotel room when the extension is used. It might be enjoyable to explore even the most normal sexual activities or positions with this extender, as the sensations could be completely new to both partners.

Let the female player give the male a "hand job" or oral sex. The male partner may find new enjoyment in watching his big new friend penetrate the female partner.

Remote Control Orgasm Game

What you need:

Is a road trip on your agenda soon? Pack a new toy—a remote control vibrator. Pack some extra batteries as well

How to Play:

Before you leave for your trip, you surprise her with a

beautifully wrapped package. She giggles and stuffs it into a bag and leaves it behind. You insist she put it on. The object of this game is to get her excited, and then bring her back down—until she is begging you to stop the car and do her—now! Tease her with it, arousing her, and then switching it off. When you get to your destination (or pull off the road into a rest area), give her an orgasm (or several) via cunnilingus.

• Start out by coordinating vibrating speed with traffic lights. When you get to a red light, give her a low buzz. On the green, accelerate.

• Or coordinate the buzz with music.

• When you come to a private rest stop, practice chivalry by opening her door, helping her out, and laying her on her back, feet up, on the front hood like a hood ornament. No privacy options? Lay her on the back seat.

• Keep the vibration on her clit for a few moments while you play in her vagina.

• Now turn off the vibe. Run a flat tongue up and down the inside of her inner lips.

• Turn your full attention to her clitoris. Tap the tip of your tongue up and down the sides. Swirl your tongue around it. Tap the tip of the clitoris.

• Suck and swirl her to orgasm.

Door-To-Door Vibrator Salesman

What you need:

You'll need a suit, briefcase, pamphlets, and, most important of all, a selection of vibrators.

How to play:

Just dress in a suit and pretend to be a door-to-door vibrator salesman. Try and surprise your lover when she thinks you're off at work or busy doing something else.

Ring the doorbell, then come into the house and explain that you have some very exciting products to show her. Take out the vibrators one by one, taking your time handling each one and explaining which are best suited for what types of play. Ask her if she'd like to borrow one and try it out (with you watching, of course)! Or for variety you can also try the one below.

Come into the house and lay down the rules: You can only show her the products if she's naked, so the first thing she has to do is strip down (or get into something comfortable, like a short and sexy bathrobe). What's more, you're going to demonstrate their effectiveness on her, whether she likes it or not. At this point, you can pull out some silk ties or handcuffs and bind her arms or legs to a chair leg. Then run through the product line one by one, taking as much time as you like to demonstrate just how effective the devices are for stimulation, teasing, and perhaps even orgasm. Ready to step it up a notch? Ask her swap roles and test the vibrators on you—maybe you'd like to try anal stimulation!

Good Vibrations

What you need:

Set a sexy scene for your night of pleasure: Build a fire, turn the lights down low, and put on some sensuous music. Have a blindfold ready and line up all your toys that vibrate, whether that's the cone, a miniature clit vibrator, or something in between.

Remember, this game is about using a variety of vibrators to tantalize every inch of your lover's body! Slowly undress your lover; kiss her deeply, and run your hands all over her body, telling her just how hot and sexy she is. Blindfold her and lead her to the vibrating pleasure zone. Start out slowly, perhaps using a vibrating wand on her neck and shoulders. Try a different vibrating device on various body parts: Massage her muscles with long smooth strokes, tickle her nipples with a vibrating finger device, and finally move to her genitals. Here you can use a vibrator to tease open her labia, switch gears to reach her G-spot, and then come back to her clitoris for the final climax!

To take it up a notch: Use a pair of vibrating nipple clips to keep her on her toes while you insert a vibrating butt plug or have her grind on a cone-like device. Once she's hot and wet, turn on that U-shaped vibrator and stimulate her G-spot and her clitoris at the same time. Let her ride the vibrations to heaven and back! Pick two or three of your favorite vibrating devices, and start at her toes. Moving very, very slowly, use each device on every inch of her, taking care to test every speed, pulsation, and pattern. Keep her guessing where you're going next and what it will feel like, and build the tension by avoiding the genitals until her clitoris is fully engorged!

Pleasure Party

What you need:

The Sexy Setup Invite your lover to a "pleasure party" designed for two. Tell him you have a special line-up of tools and tricks to bring him hours of delight. Set a sexy and

sensuous setting: Build a nest of blankets and furs on the floor, light some candles, and put on your sexiest lingerie. Line up all your sex toys, but keep them hidden under a silky scarf.

How to Play:

Welcome your lover with a long and lingering kiss, then undress him partially and ask him to get comfortable. Tell him you're the mistress of pleasure, and you're going to demonstrate all the different tools. One by one, bring out your sex toys and use them on various parts of his body, building tension and heightening the excitement as you go. Use a vibrator to massage his neck and shoulders, and then buzz his nipples gently with a vibrating finger device. Move down his body and tickle his perineum or around his testicles with your device as you stroke his penis.

Use each device to turn him on for a bit, but don't bring him to orgasm—stop and introduce the next toy until he's ready to burst! Then help him climax in whatever way feels best!

To make things hotter, help your lover undress completely, and invite him into the pleasure nest. Show him all your toys, but then blindfold him and tie his hands above his head. Tell him he must guess the toy in question as you use it on his body. If he guesses correctly, you'll reward him with a kiss (or a sip of champagne, bite of chocolate, etc.), but if he guesses incorrectly, he might get a spanking or a gentle slap. Test your toys one by one and think creatively: Use your vibrating devices on different areas of his body, slip on a cock ring and ride him for a few minutes, then jump off and insert his penis into a sleeve. Keep him guessing until he can't hold back! If you dare, try multiple toys at once: Insert a string of anal beads, and then press your bullet vibrator against the base of his penis while you suck him off. Pull out the beads just as he climaxes!

The Glory Hole

What you need:

A suction cup dildo, glory hole is defined as a small hole in a wall where the man will fit his penis in it, and the person on the other side will caress it. For this experiment, it would be good to find a dildo with a suction cup backing that will allow it to stick to a wall.

How to Play:

This may imitate the idea that another male person is remaining anonymous behind the wall and allow the two partners to play out different fantasies with the "third person."

Both partners could take turns, giving the imaginary person "head." The female partner could use the dildo to penetrate herself while she gives oral sex to the male partner. In essence, she would have control over her penetration. The male partner could also use it for anal penetration if he felt so inclined. If an added level of danger is desired, the dildo could be taken places where a glory hole might be found, such as gas stations or public restrooms or adult theatres.

Chapter 9: Advanced Sex Games for the Adventurous Couples

Maybe you and your partner have already been dabbling in sex games and are looking to kick things up another notch, or you simply want to try out some more adventurous games. Well, we've got you covered. There is research that has found that those who usually engage in new activities like sex games have higher satisfaction levels than couples who don't. Sex games help the couples have more exciting life together.

The games that we will go over will be a mixture of completely free options that will only require your imagination, while others will make you buy something. As always, make sure that you have your partner's consent before trying something new in bed.

Sexy Retail Therapy

For this one, you and your partner will head out for some shopping. You can do this in person or online. You can both pick out something that you would like to see the other one in, or one of you can pick out clothes for the other, whichever way works best for you. Once the clothes arrive, have some fun watching their jaw drop as you get dressed up.

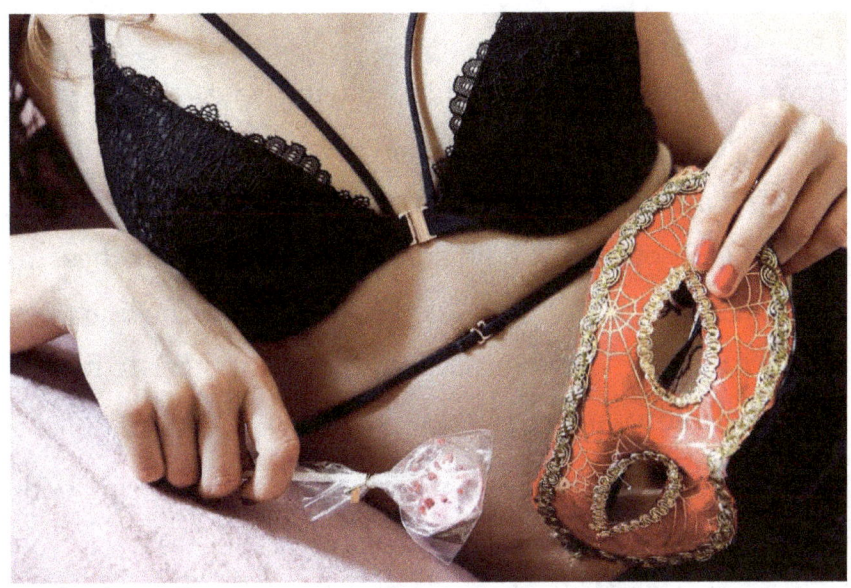

Drive and Dare

We've already talked about how a lot of people find the idea of doing something kinky outdoors or in public is hot. So this game lets you get freaky al fresco. To play this game, both of you need to put on some skimpy clothes. It could be a sexy black dress or some flimsy shorts and a simple t-shirt. Then go drive for a while. You will take turns suggesting places to that you will stop at. When you make a stop, the person who chose the place will be dared by his or her partner to go out and do some naughty things.

Keep the dared low-key to make sure you don't draw a lot of attention to yourself. Then when you start to make the trip back home, start to move your hand up your partner's leg to let them know you want do something together.

Tear It Up

Have you ever fantasized about having wild, rip off your clothes sex, but didn't want to mess up your own clothes? Then you are going to want to try this game. All you have to do is head out and buy some super-cheap clothes. A secondhand store may be a good option. Wash them up, get dressed, and then let your partner know that they are free to rip them to shreds.

There is a lot of other ways to tear it up. You can both unleash your carnal lust and have a rip-fest, or you incorporate the ripping into a points-based game. It is all up to you. If you love having rough sex, then you are going to love this.

Strip Pong

This takes beer pong to a whole new level. Clear off your dining table and then place six plastic cups in the form of atriangle. Fill up the cups with beer or your favorite alcohol and then take turns trying to toss a ping pong ball into the other person's cups. When a person scores, their partner has to down what is in the cup that the ball landed in and then take off a clothing. The person who first gets a ball in to all 6 cups will get to ask for something special.

Toy Tease Time

While retail therapy is all about looks, this game gives you the chance to try out the toys you have fantasized about. Again, you can go to a sex store in person or shop online, but purchase some sex toys that you have always wanted to try out. Don't worry if you don't know where to start. To add more fun to this game, make a list of what you have always wanted to try and give it to your partner. They can then buy whichever ones they want that are on that list. Once the items arrive, you can play a little game. You will be blindfolded and on the bed, and your partner will pull out the toys, one at a time, and gently tease you with them. If you are able to guess what it is in three guesses, then they will bring you to orgasm with it.

Position Challenge

If you would like to have a game that will also make sex last longer, this is the best game. The main objective of the game is a simple one, see how many different positions that two of you can do in one sex session before you both reach orgasm. This game will improve the more often you do it, as you can try to top what you did last time.

Seven Minutes in Heaven

Have you ever gotten to enjoy the excitement of trying to squeeze in a quickie before somebody comes in and finds out? This is the game that will help you to recapture that thrill of having only a certain amount of time to do it. Get a timer and set you and your partner a limit of seven minutes. Then find yourself space, like a closet, and see if the two of you can bang out a quickie before your time is up. This can be a thrilling and fun game to bring the two of you closer together.

House Party

The party is all about holding off an orgasm. Nobody can climax until you have banged in every single room in your house. That's all you have to do is try to have sex in each room before you both climax. You can also use this game as a form of foreplay.

The Oral Master

If your foreplay game seems to be lacking, then you could try the oral master game. All you need to do is set a timer for four minutes and see who is able to initiate the most oral sex positions before time is up. Make sure that you keep score, and then you can swap roles to discover who the master of oral sex is. This also gives you the chance to learn a few more oral sex positions, especially if your knowledge has been limited to a kneeling blow job.

Orgasm Race

This game is all about mutual masturbation and is the best game to try to help bring you and your partner closer. Since most people masturbate by themselves, doing that in front of somebody else will heighten your sense of vulnerability and will help to increase your intimacy. This will also allow you to show your partner exactly what it is that you like and how you want it.

In order to have an orgasm race, you will like beside one another and start pleasuring each other. Whichever person climaxes first is the winner and will continue to pleasure their partner until they climax. You can also set the stipulation that thin winner gets to request a sexy little treat the next time you do it.

Name the Letter

This is another game that can spice up your oral sex and foreplay. This game is a great way to explore the body of your partner. All you need to do is have them lie down, blindfold them, and then pick your favorite part on them, like their genitals, breasts, or tummy. Then you will gently form a letter onto their skin, making sure you keep the movements teasing and light. If they guess the letter right, they receive one point. Once they get 10 correct response, they get an orgasm, and so you will swap places.

Put It in My Mouth

If you are really looking to up your desire levels, nothing beats the combo of sex and food. In order to play this, get naked, blindfold your partner, and then they will feed you some delicious foods. You can pick out any of your favorite foods, but sweet foods are typically the best when paired with sex, such as strawberries, yogurt, ice cream, cake, or, the classic, chocolate.

Since your partner is blindfolded, the spoon is going to wind up in several places. And there is one simple rule, whatever gets spilled on you, they have to lick it off. You can guide them toward the right spots. This is an amazing game for trust-building, and you are going to love the sensation of having the food licked off of your body.

Chapter 10:   Sex Games with Drinks

It Takes Two to Tango

When we come to the point of talking about alcoholic drinks and sex games, one can't resist the opportunity to think about the different classic hot sex games you can do. To start, one just needs to have an empty bottle; it can be a bottle of your preferred alcohol.

Simply turn the bottle around and act out the one being asked for. When the bottle points to your partner, different types of kiss must be given to you. Also, in the event that you need to add somewhat more flavor to the game, you can utilize whipped cream or chocolate spread which of course will depend on what flavor you preferred and if the end of the bottle points to your partner, he must lick it from your body and indulge in whatever food you chose to heighten up the sexual anticipation.

Sexy Coin Toss or Heads or Butts

The classic game of coin toss is transformed into a hot, sexy and dirty version that couples will love. At each flip of the coin, both of you must bet opposite, guessing if it will heads or butts. The one fails to think it correctly must drink one shot and take off one piece of clothing they have on. The games end when one of you is already fully naked, which will then pave the way to more hot and sexy foreplay.

Boozy Body Shots

One of the most classic and straightforward sexy booze games, all you need to have would be two pieces of dice, pen and paper, shot glasses and your favorite alcohol. Write on the part of the paper the different areas of the body and fold them, and indicate a number for each piece of paper. The player will then throw the dice and get the corresponding numbered paper. Whatever body part is written is where the shot of booze must be taken from.

Straight Face Is the Game

Provide both of you and your partner a piece of paper, each where you will list 6-12 naughty, dirty and erotic words you can think of without revealing them to one another.

Once done, fold each cut piece of paper and toss them into a bowl. With each turn, you and your partner will take one piece of paper and try to recite it so anyone can hear without showing even a bit of emotion. In the event that you and your partner can keep a straight face, no consequence will be served. Among the two of you, the one who will show a pinch of emotion, a grin, laugh or cringe must take one shot.

Hot Vodka Twister

Balance is the main concept of the game Twister, and adding the element of getting drunk will make it more exciting and way more fun. Play the game the usual way, but to make it different, put several vodka shots and some glasses with water on the sheet's number. After spinning, drink the shot on the number before you put your leg or hand on it. Lucky for you, if you drink a shot of water. All this drinking, touching and getting close to each other's body will inevitably end up in the bedroom afterward.

Steamy Eye Contact Game (Don't Blink Or Else)

Here's your chance to look into each other's eyes deeply without getting awkward. While looking into each other's eye, you must be still and prevent your eyes from blinking. The one who blinks will need to take a shot and strip off one piece of garment. This game will heighten the feeling of sexual anticipation and tension between the two of you. Maybe you can wear provocative clothes, so you'll make it more difficult for them to concentrate looking into your eyes.

Body Treasure Map (X Marks the Spot)

If you are looking for a chance and a reason to kiss your love, now is the best timing for that. In this game, your main goals are to remember where you want to be kissed and licked with their lips and tongue. Give your partner 4 chances in guessing where your preferred X spot is. If they are correct in guessing, then lucky for you because you'll be receiving some kissed and licking on that spot, but if they were not able to guess, they have to take 3 shots of your chosen alcohol. Keep playing, guessing and kissing all you want until the both of you are horny and drunk to finish it off in the bedroom.

Striptease Q&A

The first step in this game is for you to think of one word, may it be a thing, person, place, animal or emotion. Don't reveal the word to your partner yet. Give them 3 chances in guessing the word and let them ask you questions that you can answer with a yes and no for them to have clues. For each question they ask, they must give an answer, and if it wrong, your partner must take a shot and kiss you somewhere you like. If, in the end, they were not able to give the word, your partner must do lap dance and striptease for you, and of course, you know what comes next.

Blinded Erotic Touch

Blindfolds are known as one of the most erotic things you can use in doing foreplay and seduction. The reason behind this can be that when other senses are blocked, the remaining senses will be more sensitive. All feelings will be intensified, and a simple touch before will feel more intense when blindfolded. Having said this, if you want to make your next drinking session an erotic one, this game is something you must do. The first step is to have one of you blindfolded, then one who isn't will act as the guide and put the index finger on several areas of the body (better if its the erogenous zones) The once who has blindfold must then guess which body part are they touching. If your partner doesn't give the correct body part, he must take a shot, but if he does, you are the one who needs to take a shot.

Chapter 11:   Truth or Dare and Would You Rather Sex Games

Truth or Dare

If you and your partner like to be naughty when it comes to truth or dares then this is the part for you.

There are three ways to use the information in this.

First, you can use the following requests and questions you can use to supplement your games. In case you run out of things to say or your mind goes blank, you can just flip to this and you have an entire archive of what to say.

Second, you can use this directly to engage in a deeply sexual and arousing conversation.

Finally, you can actually print this andcut them out as little cards and drop them into a bowl that you can draw out of later.

1.   What, if done right before orgasm, will make it one of the best you've ever had?

2.   Kiss your way down the front of my neck, down through my crotch, and then back up my spine.

3.   Perform oral sex on my hand and show me exactly how you like it.

4.   In what circumstances would you prefer to skip

foreplay?

5.   Would you prefer to be completely silent or incredibly loud during sex?

6.   What turns you on to see in public?

7.   Show me how you would try to seduce me into bed for the first time.

8.   Would you have sex with me in a dressing room or public restroom?

9.   Go into the next room and you have 2 minutes to take 3 sexy photos. Send them to me.

10.   Where would you most like to have sex that we have not yet?

11.   Take a picture of us kissing passionately.

12.   What is your most embarrassing moment during sex?

13.   Film yourself orgasming for me tomorrow before noon.

14.   What dirty talk phrase immediately turns you on?

15.   Tell me about our last sexual encounter in as much detail as possible.

16.   Do anything you want with me for the next 60 seconds.

17.   What position or act would you like to do more of?

18.   Kiss me for 40 seconds.

19. What do you like to hear me say during sex?

20. Nibble your name onto my back and neck.

21. Nibble my ears for 20 seconds each.

22. Describe what it's like to have sex with me.

23. Put a blindfold on me and run a feather or piece of cloth across my bare chest and thighs.

24. Begin touching yourself and continue for the remainder of this game.

25. Make your mouth hot with a warm liquid and then give oral.

26. Make your mouth cold with ice and then give oral.

27. Reenact a random porn scene you find right now by going to Pornhub, typing a random letter, and then choosing the 8th video.

28. Download a Kama Sutra app on your phone and find three positions you want to try next time.

29. Eat a banana in the sexiest way possible and keep a straight face.

30. Act like a submissive for the next 2 minutes.

31. Act like a master/dom for the next 2 minutes.

32. Strip naked and take a walk around the block.

33. Groom my pubic region.

34. Put Icy Hot or Ben Gay on your nipples.

35. Give me a hickey on my ass cheek.

36. Pretend to have a VERY loud and intense orgasm.

37. Name all the sex toys you have ever used.

38. What is the shortest amount of time it can take you to orgasm?

39. Drip honey (or chocolate or anything else) onto my chest and lick it off.

40. Give me a 3 minute massage.

41. If you could receive anything sex-related as a present, what would it be?

42. Let's reenact a piece of written erotica right now.

43. Would you rather have sex with someone watch, or watch people have sex?

44. Which Disney character or cartoon is most sexually attractive to you?

45. No underwear for the rest of the day for you.

46. Do a cartwheel naked.

47. What is your favorite type of porn?

48. When did you last masturbate?

49. What is the first thing you would do if you could

change genders for a day?

50. Would you prefer: a partner with a horrible body but great face, or great body and horrible face?

51. Switch clothing – whatever fits.

52. Show me the most sensitive part of your body.

53. What is your sexual brag about your abilities?

54. Describe exactly how your orgasms feel.

55. What would your stripper theme song be?

56. Unwrap a piece of candy in your mouth.

57. Both of you will take your bottoms off and start spooning immediately.

58. Drip ice water over your partner's naked body.

59. Drip candle wax over your partner's naked chest.

60. Give five minutes of oral right now.

Would You Rather Questions
WOULD YOU RATHER...

Have sex with the person you hate the most

Or

Have sex with a homeless guy?

WOULD YOU RATHER...

Suck an old but clean guy

Or

Have sex with the person you love but he or she didn't take a shower since 5 months?

WOULD YOU RATHER...

Fuck someone of your family one time

Or

Never be able to have sex with someone for your life?

WOULD YOU RATHER...

Lick a pussy

Or

Lick an asshole?

WOULD YOU RATHER...

Live with a sexy girl/guy but be only allowed to kiss him/her

Or

Live with an ugly man/woman but you can have sex anytime you want?

WOULD YOU RATHER...

Lick the feet of someone you hate for 1 million dollars

Or

Be able to kick the ass of this same person for free without any problem?

WOULD YOU RATHER...

Have butt sex

Or

be sucked or licked?

WOULD YOU RATHER...

Have sex with every person who ask you even if you don't want

Or

Never have sex again?

WOULD YOU RATHER...

Stay one crazy night with 2 very sexy girls/guys but you can fuck with them only one hour

Or

Stay one week with a basic girl/guy but you can fuck with her/him every hour?

WOULD YOU RATHER...

Suck/lick your best friend

Or

Be sucked/licked by your best friend?

WOULD YOU RATHER...

Casual sex

Or

Hardcore sex?

WOULD YOU RATHER...

Have sex with 2 girls and 1 guy

Or

Have sex with 2 guys and 1 girl?

WOULD YOU RATHER...

Have a sex slave

Or

Become a sex slave?

WOULD YOU RATHER...

Make a French kiss with your dad

Or

Lick the ass of a homeless guy?

WOULD YOU RATHER...

Have sex with a Japanese guy/girl

Or

A Latina/Latino?

WOULD YOU RATHER...

Earn 10 000 $ per month without working

Or

Be able to have sexy with everyone you want when you want?

WOULD YOU RATHER...

Lick a stranger foot

Or

Lick a subway seat?

WOULD YOU RATHER...

Have sex in the subway with a beautiful girl

Or

Have sex with a casual girl in a bed?

WOULD YOU RATHER...

Lick your sister's nipples

Or

Lick your brother's dick?

WOULD YOU RATHER...

Suck a dick every time you say something stupid

Or

Be fucked every time you say something smart?

WOULD YOU RATHER...

Blow your friend but no one knows about that

Or

Don't do it but everyone think you did it?

WOULD YOU RATHER...

save your boyfriend/girlfriend but you have to suck the dick of a dog

Or

Didn't save him/her?

WOULD YOU RATHER...

your boyfriend/girlfriend cheats on you

Or

You cheat on your boyfriend/girlfriend?

WOULD YOU RATHER...

Your boyfriend/girlfriend pee in your mouth

Or

You have to lick his/her mom pussy instead?

WOULD YOU RATHER...

Lick sperm on a public toilet seat

Or

Lick a grandma toe?

WOULD YOU RATHER...

Your boyfriend/girlfriend have sex with someone else but thinking about you at the same time

Or

You have sex with your boyfriend/girlfriend but (s)he's thinking about someone else?

WOULD YOU RATHER...

Lick an Us Marine foot after 48 hours on the field

Or

Lick a firefighter dirty armpit?

WOULD YOU RATHER...

Doggy Style

Or

Missionary position?

WOULD YOU RATHER...

Have sex in a public place

Or

Have sex in a plane?

WOULD YOU RATHER...

Have a sex in a black room

Or

Have sex with a black person?

WOULD YOU RATHER...

watch your mom in a gang bang

Or

Take her place?

WOULD YOU RATHER...

Be a slave

Or

A master?

WOULD YOU RATHER...

Have sex with a very dirty stranger

Or

With someone in your family?

WOULD YOU RATHER...

Have sex with the sexiest actor/actress in the world

Or

With an anime character of your choice?

WOULD YOU RATHER...

Watch the sex tape of your parents

Or

Make a sex tape in a public space in front of 100 persons?

WOULD YOU RATHER...

Lick a dirty asshole of a very sexy girl/guy

Or

Lick a clean asshole of a very ugly guy/girl?

WOULD YOU RATHER...

Drink one liter of sperm in 1 week

Or

10 liter of diet coke in the same day?

WOULD YOU RATHER...

Give your little sister to a pervert guy for 1 day

Or

Go with this guy for 1 week and you have to do everything he wants?

WOULD YOU RATHER...

Going on vacations with 10 sexy girls but you can only kiss them

Or

With one ugly girl but she does everything you want?

WOULD YOU RATHER...

Lick the hairy balls of a very handsome guy

Or

Have a French kiss with an ugly guy?

WOULD YOU RATHER...

Have a romance with Ryan Gosling for 10 years but you have to suck Donald Trump dick every time he wants for 1 week

Or

The opposite?

WOULD YOU RATHER...

Suck a donkey dick

Or

Be fucked on a doggy style by a dog?

WOULD YOU RATHER...

Walk naked in the middle of Time Square for 10 minutes

Or

Run 10 km naked in the snow in the middle of nowhere?

WOULD YOU RATHER...

Lick the pole to stand in the subway

Or

Kiss a stranger in the street?

WOULD YOU RATHER...

Have sex with a Korean Girl/Guy

Or

With a French Girl/Guy?

WOULD YOU RATHER...

Have sex with 3 girls and 1 guy

Or

With 2 girls and 2 guys?

WOULD YOU RATHER...

Never use Internet again

Or

Never have sex again?

WOULD YOU RATHER...

Lick the underwear of someone else

Or

Use the toothbrush of someone else?

WOULD YOU RATHER...

Eat a cockroach alive

Or

Lick the armpit of a homeless guy?

WOULD YOU RATHER...

Must kiss every butt of people you meet for life

Or

have a French kiss with everyone you meet?

Chapter 12:   Excellent Tips to Blow Your Partner's Mind in Bed

Investing time in learning the teachings of this book can help you provide mind-blowing orgasms to your partner. It can be very difficult for some people to reach orgasm but when you have the skills you need it can be achieved quite easily. There are some major components to ensuring that somebody can reach orgasm. In terms of a woman, they need to be extremely comfortable in their situation should be able to climax. Men are a little bit easier when it comes to this area; however, sometimes it can be difficult for them as well.

Obviously, the tips and tricks that you will use to ensure your lady has a mind-blowing orgasm are going to be quite different than the ones to ensure that the male counterpart is getting his. There are different tactics that are going to be used in different situations. It does not have to be difficult to ensure that your partner reaches orgasm as long as you have the information and ability to do it. Let's take a look at both sexes and what you can do to ensure that they have mind-blowing orgasm's each and every time you participate in a sexual encounter.

We're going to start off by looking at the ladies. There are a

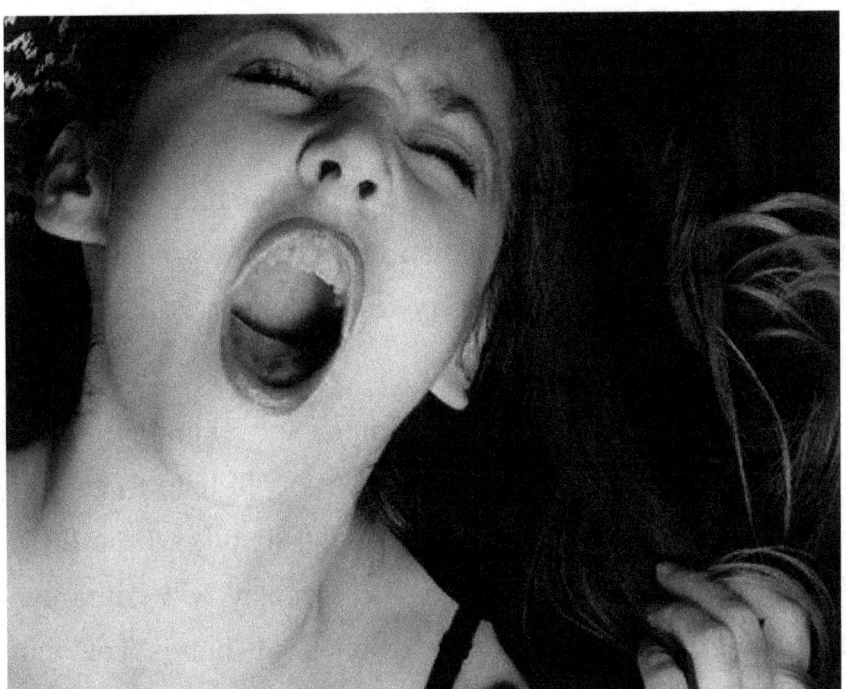

variety of different things you can do to make it easier for her to achieve an orgasm. Most women admit that they have faked a few orgasms in their life. Unfortunately, a few is a gross understatement for how many times most women have faked it. It is unfortunate that they believe that they need to do this to make their sexual partners feel satisfied. Men, you must remember that you can't pressure a woman into having an orgasm. It is something that is going to take time and honestly, there are going to be times she absolutely cannot get there. This is OK as the experience of sexual intimacy is fulfilling enough during those times that orgasm cannot be achieved.

The environment that you put your lady and will play a big role as to whether or not she is going to be able to climax. As noted, women need to feel comfortable and relaxed to be able to have an orgasm. So, setting the mood for your woman is more important than ever if you want to ensure that she has an orgasm every time you enter into sexual intercourse.

We cannot iterate enough how important taking your time and investing it in 4 play is. This tactic will help to get her warm before actual intercourse begins. It takes time for a lady to become truly aroused and foreplay will guarantee that she is. Using your mouth in your hands you can stimulate all of her erogenous zones and have her reeling when it's time actually to penetrate her.

You need to keep in mind that for most women it can take an average of about 20 minutes for them to achieve climax. So, when a man ejaculates prior to this it can be very frustrating for the woman. If you cannot last longer to provide her with the time, she needs to climax don't leave her stranded. You can pleasure her after you have reached orgasm to ensure that she also gets hers. It can be a little bit messy, but she will certainly appreciate it if you decide to slide in a couple of fingers to finish her off after you have climaxed.

Another great tip for ensuring that your lady reaches orgasm is to focus on her clitoris. Most women cannot achieve orgasm from simple penetration. The combination of penetration and clitoral stimulation is utterly amazing from the female's perspective. In fact, most women would rather you simply focus on their clitoris to help them achieve climax. Penetration is fantastic and most women enjoy it; however, it is likely not going to be enough to get her there truly.

You also want to make sure to encourage dirty talk. Being naughty before and during intercourse can be truly stimulating. It turns women on and allows them to relax. Most women do not want to participate in a sexual encounter with an extremely shy man. So, be bold and open your mouth to state all of your wants and desires. She will truly appreciate it.

Last but not least, work on finding her G-spot. Yes, the G-spot actually exists. It is typically located a couple of inches inside of her vagina on the front wall. With a little bit of pressure and a circular pattern of movement, you can stimulate her G-spot. This can lead to female ejaculation and some of the best orgasms she has ever experienced in her life. If you add to that some clitoral stimulation you will seriously be driving her wild.

Now that we've looked at a few things that men can do to

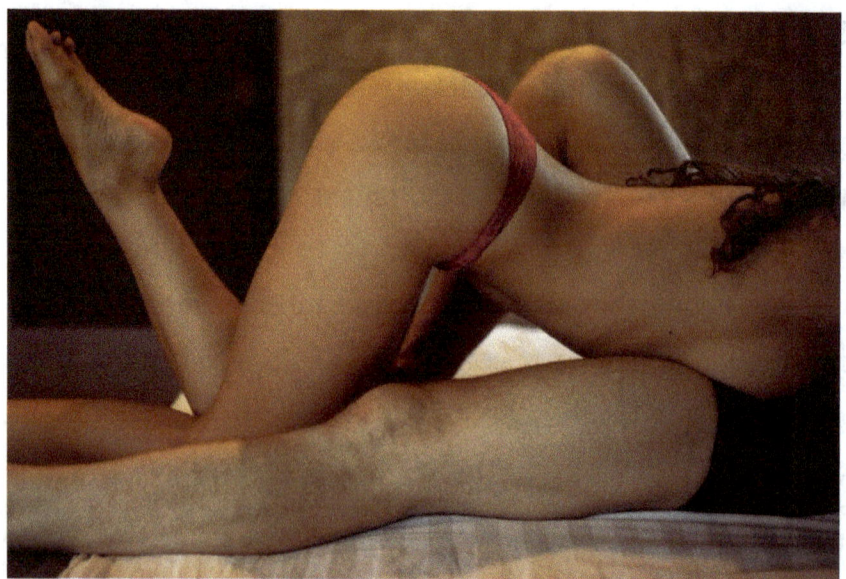

ensure that their ladies have amazing orgasm's let's reverse the role. Figuring out exactly what to do to ensure that he has a mind-blowing orgasm can seem intimidating for some people. This is especially true if you are lacking in, experience. Keep in mind that sex is a learning process and you will get better the more that you do it. In addition, the more you know your partner is the better level of communication you have the easier it will be to do the things that truly please them.

While it may be easier to give your man an orgasm than it is for him to give you one you need to realize that there are definitely different levels. Some orgasms for men are simply OK while others are completely off the charts. Obviously, we want to provide our male counterparts with orgasm's that are consistently off the charts. Let's look at some different techniques that can help you accomplish this.

Just like women, men need to be relaxed and undistracted to achieve orgasm. So, setting the mood can be advantageous in helping them push their daily stresses out of their minds and focus on the intimacy that is about to commence. In addition, foreplay is almost as important to men as it is to women. This ramp-up. It allows the sexual tension to heighten and make intercourse much more stimulating.

When intimacy is done right both partners are focused on each other. Oftentimes, this leads to a man pushing off his orgasm until his female counterpart has been satisfied. One way to ensure that your man has a mind-blowing orgasm is to tell him he doesn't need to worry about you. Make the sexual session all about him. Allow him to lay back while you take control. Encourage him to climax whenever he can even if it is quickly. This can be very freeing for a partner and reduced their level of worry which, in turn, will allow them to have a mind-blowing orgasm.

Another great piece of advice that can help your man have a mind-blowing orgasm is to withhold it for a few days. Yes, this can be difficult for both parties. It is especially true if you have an exceptionally sexual relationship. By denying actual intercourse you can really ramp both parties up to have seriously intense orgasms. It will take a bit of willpower; however, you will both be appreciative in the end.

One other tip that can help your man achieve a mind-blowing orgasm is to surprise him. In the afternoon quickie is not something most women initiate. However, it is something that should be initiated more frequently. Surprising him with a random tumble in the sheets it can really heighten his level of pleasure and the experience he has during intercourse.

As with all things, the tips that we have given you to help heighten the level of orgasm for your partner are only a few of the many things that work. If you have tried all of these things continue to do some research as there are more options out there. Simply trying to ensure that your partner is achieving excellent orgasms is a step in the right direction and the more you try the more successful you will be.

Conclusion

Sex is beautiful, the result of passion and alchemy. Especially in couples, when love and creativity present a beautiful moment of sensuality in life. But over time, the flame fades and something needs to be done to maintain it. Especially after a long life together, involving birthdays, discussions, children, work and economic problems, illness, long-term household and daily affairs, and law, many couples are often plagued by questions about how to find and restore that passion. This fire, the sexual desire that marked the first years of their relationship.

Monotony can kill passion, and anyone who lives in a sexless marriage knows that this statement is entirely true. Sex and passion can be removed from any situation that leads to routine, so that even a long relationship, even if it is not sealed by a marriage relationship, is not free from that risk.

Monotonous daily life, stress, fatigue from a life that is not always easy, and the problems of daily life can cause a partner's intimate life to be in the background and have more or less important implications for stability. If all these cases occur, or at some point in marriage, the physiological decline of desire occurs and sex is a distant memory that is conscious of what is happening and tries to maintain mentality, it will seriously ask how and with what strategy

Reacting is reproductive passion and desire.

Causes can be physical or psychological, such as stress, depression, fatigue, anxiety, involvement and lack of time. First of all, you have to ask yourself whether this always happens, or whether reluctance to take initiative is new to the relationship. Conversely, if you find that after you always want to make love, but the desire has fallen asleep from time to time, this can be a moment of normal use, a deeper problem. Over time, a slight decrease in partner's libido is normal, but we don't have to be discouraged, sex can and should continue to be an important attachment for couples.

Even in the elderly, desires can be easily maintained in healthy subjects. Therefore, it is important to understand the causes of shared problems and find the right solution. Clean sensuality by sleeping during the routine.

1. Dialogue, talk about your decline, even if you feel uncomfortable. Remembering this thorny object, with the right words and without blaming anyone, the fruit is seen. You must be open and honest. If there is a problem, if something is wrong - even from a sexual point of view - speaking openly is the first and perhaps most effective way to resolve the situation. It is important that you talk to each other after you have minimal self-reflection so that you clearly explain to your partner what problems need to be

addressed. When you stop talking to other, problems accumulate and are unresolved, with consequences we can imagine.

2. Teasing shamelessly. Play, find the things that inspire you the most, make passion not a marriage assignment, but a pleasant pleasure.

3. Satisfy your partner's frustrated fantasy. If a partner always wants to have something definite in sex and is never "happy," the moment of arousal can be the right person to try to satisfy. Obviously, you don't have to do things that you don't want or don't want to do. If this is possible, this choice of avenue can open the door to a new dimension for intimate life and life as a couple.

4. Take time for weekly sexual encounters. This might look a little sexy, but in the opinion of many researchers the best choice. That way you can make it funny, different, and fun.

5. Intimacy is not just about having sex. Find connections to your partner without having to request an all-inclusive package. Massage and hugs, caresses and kisses help intimacy, and not directly.

6. Consider the past. Try to find the best period of activity in your sex life and look for its characteristics. Talk about it and let them understand what you missed and what other parts of the apple want.

7. Surprise effect. If you eat pasta or pizza every day because you like it, it's only natural that you get rejected after a month. Try something new. If long-term relationship problems focus on boredom and everyday life, there's nothing better than trying new things and exploring unknown areas. It is enough to offer something new, but also to surprise your partner (maybe in underwear more than usual) to take the attitude that the couple would not expect.

8. Sensuality outside the home. Arrange special meetings: a walk on the beach, a fireplace with background music, a very sexy dinner, a steam bath. However, there might be sex without love, but there is no love without sex.

9. Find your personal moments. It is a good idea to save at least one or two hours a week to devote yourself to your partner, even if you are recovering from everyday stress, talk about dreams and hopes and rely on each other to find closeness and compassion in risk. Also it helps to go out any time or to take short breaks, a relaxing day or a romantic weekend. Affective intimacy is also an important factor for happy relationships in sexual matters. A good couple trip will be enough to spend the weekend. It could be ideal a weekend at a spa that combines a revival of passion with relaxation and well-being together.

10. Sex quality. With increasing age and involvement, decreased sexual activity is almost "physiological", but quality and quantity are often confused. In fact, frequency is not the most important factor to fulfill sex life. Better is rare, but better than frequent and fast.

The daily application of sensitive and receptive behaviors in long-term partners can increase male and female sexual understanding and desire, especially if this particular attitude gives a partner a sense of value. Understanding the needs of others, both through emotional affirmation and through listening, closeness and affection, increases sexual desire, especially when those feelings give the impression that the other person is valuable and that sexual relations with a partner are highly desirable.

CPSIA information can be obtained
at www.ICGtesting.com
Printed in the USA
BVHW052033080521
606756BV00004B/806